Play as if Your Life Depends on It

functional exercise and living for *Homo sapiens*

Frank Forencich

ISBN 0-9723358-0-3

Library of Congress Control Number: 2002093564

Printed in the United States of America

Before the High and Far-Off Times, O my
Best Beloved, came the Time of the Very
Beginnings; and that was in the days when the
Eldest Magician was getting Things ready. First
he got the Earth ready; then he got the Sea
ready; and then he told all the Animals that
they could come out and play.

Rudyard Kipling

The Crab That Played with the Sea

People are beginning to see that the first requisite
to success in life is to be a good animal.

Herbert Spencer

Contents

Warm-up

Being a creature of obvious intelligence, good judgment and curiosity, you've no doubt spent some time wondering about the human body and how it works. Perhaps you've studied some physiology and picked up a few things about exercise and nutrition. You've played a few sports and sampled a variety of training practices. Maybe you're an athlete, a trainer, a coach, a physical therapist or a physical educator. Maybe you're already a supremely fit warrior-athlete or maybe you're struggling to get back in shape after a long layoff.

In any case, you've had some good physical experiences, but at the same time, something seems incomplete. Perhaps the fitness world isn't giving you what you thought it would. Maybe your motivation is flagging or you're suffering from some kind of activity-related injury. Maybe you've got the desire, but you just can't find an exercise program that works for you.

We all want to get in shape, that's clear enough, but we're also looking for meaning and depth in the process. Many of us are looking for particular changes and improvements to our bodies, but we also suspect that there's more to physical training than just sets, reps and mileage. We're looking for something that's relevant to the totality of our lives, something that is satisfying, substantive and sustainable. Not only that, we're looking for something that's interesting, exciting and fun.

When we look into the world of exercise, we find that there is plenty of information out there about fitness. We see dozens of books on strength training, weight-loss, aerobics, stretching and every sport imaginable. Lots of this information is up-to-date, accurate and well-researched. It's safe to say that there we now have more information available on fitness than at any time in human history. If information was the solution to our physical problems, we'd be in great condition by now.

The problem is that most of these books treat the body in isolation. Typically, they look at one particular facet of human physiology, exercise or performance. They present information about weight-loss, nutrition, strength, flexibility or single-sport per-formance, completely ignoring the historical reality and evolution of the human body. In fact, many of these books treat the body as if it simply fell from the sky one sunny afternoon, independent and completely without history or context.

We similar characteristics in popular exercise programs. As it stands, the fitness industry consists of a bewildering jumble of programs and certification organizations. By some counts, there are as many as 250 fitness organizations, many of which have their own standards for training and certification. There are certificates for weight management, weight training, aerobics, yoga, martial arts, taebo, jazzercise, spinning, water exercise, senior classes and a whole host of disease-specific programs. And yet, not one of these programs connects its instructional content with human evolution or our heritage as hunters and gatherers.

But as you will see, the human body has an immensely deep biological history, a history that has shaped every detail of our physiology. This heritage has profound implications for how we might shape our exercise and conditioning programs. It suggests ways to exercise that are not only appropriate for our bodies, but pleasurable as well. While it is possible to study human physiology and fitness without looking at our evolutionary heritage, we can do much better if we take our history into account. By looking back to our origins, we can discover ways to improve our health, sharpen our performance and give a deeper sense of meaning to our physical practices. If a fitness program is to be compelling and sustainable, it has to be holistic. And if it's going to be holistic, it has to offer some connection to primal human experience and the deep history of our bodies.

As we grope our way into the 21st century, it is becoming increas-ingly obvious that many of us are suffering ill health and that much of it can be traced directly back to inactivity and sedentary living. It is also becoming clear that our current programs and orientations towards physical fitness simply aren't working. It's time that we re-examined the core concepts behind exercise and if necessary, create a new orientation from scratch. This is what we'll try to do in this book.

The orientation that you'll find in these pages comes in large measure from my own personal effort to find some congruence between human biology and physical training. As a physical omnivore, I've participated in a wide range of sport and movement disciplines; martial art, climbing, trail running and not surprisingly, physical rehabilitation. As a teacher of movement and exercise, I have been forced to examine the objectives and philosophies that underlie various training practices. When I wasn't actually training, I was reading broadly in biology, evolution and anthropology, desperately trying to reconcile my physical practices with recent discoveries about human origins.

After two decades of study, struggle and experimentation I've come to the conclusion that what we need is a paradigm for human fitness that meets a few simple conditions: it's got to have some relevance to human origins, it's got to speak to the functional performance of the human body and it's got to be fun. In other words, we need a paradigm for exercise and fitness that's primal, practical and playful.

As you'll discover, these three principles fit together in an overlapping, interdependent and complementary fashion. Each reinforces the other to form a complete, integrated approach to physical fitness and living. By studying these perspectives, you'll be able to create a personal fitness program that is both satisfying and sustainable. In the process, you'll gain a fresh enthusiasm for movement and your body.

primal

The primal comes first. If we're going to get back into shape, we'll need to revisit our origins and relearn the basic movements that brought us here in the first place. We don't need a higher education in exercise science; we need a lower education in primal human movement. We don't need more fitness data and tips, we need more experience and participation, especially experience that is consistent with our evolutionary history.

In large measure, this book is built on one foundational assumption: by choosing exercises and training practices that are consistent with human evolution, we will be more likely to get results, avoid injury and have fun in the process. Human physiology and biomechanics have been sculpted over the course of millions of years to enhance our survival in a semi-wooded grassland environment. If we can mimic those challenges, even in some small measure, we'll increase the probability of improving our health and fitness.

My goal is to stimulate your imagination and get you thinking about your ancestral heritage and what it means for your physical life. I'll ask you to imagine your days and nights on the African plain, how you would move, what you would see and feel. As you will see, imagination is a crucial part of a physical fitness program.

Don't get the wrong idea. It's not that we need to duplicate the exact conditions of human evolution in our physical training practices. I won't suggest that you live naked in the bush, sleep on the ground or subsist on a diet of insects. Instead, I will encourage you to develop an orientation towards our ancestral physicality. We need games and exercises that have some plausible relevance to human evolution. The idea is to mimic those physical challenges that we have adapted to over the course of millions of years. For this, we'll need some knowledge of ancestral conditions and the imagination to put it into a modern practice.

This book is based in large measure on the idea that knowledge of human evolution can tell us something important about modern bodies and behaviors. This kind of evolutionary reasoning is becoming increasingly popular in many body-related disciplines. We are now seeing the widespread application of evolutionary knowledge in fields such as medicine, psychology, neurology and nutrition: it is inevitable that exercise will be studied in the same light.

Of course, there is a certain amount of speculation involved in extrapolating from ancestral conditions to modern living. We can't say for certain that mimicking the physical challenges of our deep past will cure our physical woes. Duplicating primal conditions won't necessarily extend your lifespan, prevent disease or give you the body you've always wanted. Nevertheless, there is substantial explanatory power here that demands our attention. When we realize that 99% of our history was spent on the grassland and a mere 1% in modern conditions, we start to pay attention. Six million years of evolution makes a pretty compelling case.

practical

The second principle for building an effective and enjoyable physical training program is that it should be practical. The training should be simple, inexpensive and customizable for individual needs. It should be adaptable so that we can perform it in a variety of locations. Most of all, it should be functional.

Functional exercise is a paradigm for human movement that stresses performance over cosmetics and locomotion over appearance. The functional coach says, "I don't care what you look like, just as long as you can move smoothly, powerfully, effectively and without pain." This emphasis on functionality is now commonly accepted in the physical therapy community, but stands in marked contrast to the cosmetic orientation that most gyms and magazines promote.

Functional performance is the ability to execute graceful and effective movement. It is the ability to walk, sit, run, carry, jump and lift without excess fatigue or injury. In this style of training, the cosmetic appearance of the body is not particularly important. What is important is how well we move. The quality of our movement determines not only how well we perform in our occupations and recreation, but also our resistance to injury and how well we heal. It also determines our level of pleasure in the process; high quality movement is fun, rewarding and self-reinforcing.

As you study this functional orientation, it's quite likely that you'll want to know something about the relationship between functional movement and physical appearance. Obviously, a lot of us want to lose weight and look better. But as you probably know, weight management is not something that happens over the course of a few days or weeks, but consistently, month after month, year after year. To manage our weight, we've got to keep moving with a fairly regular frequency throughout our lives.

If we start by emphasizing functional performance, we build a foundation for long-term physical activity, injury-resistance and sustainability. We'll have the strength and skill to keep moving consistently, year in and year out. If you train yourself to become more functional–physically and otherwise–you'll be able to dance and play more often and more vigorously, and you won't be so worried about hurting yourself in the process. You'll be able to do more things and enjoy them more.

Eventually, if we concentrate on function, cosmetics will take care of themselves. For the most part, people who function well also look good. The form–lean, toned muscles–follows function–agility, strong legs and core body power. If you put form ahead of function, you are likely to wind up with neither. If you put function ahead of form, you will ultimately get both.

playful

The third principle is that the ideal physical training program should be playful. We don't really need much justification here, but if you want one, you can point to the fact that playful movements tend to promote balance, coordination, useful strength, speed and skill. Playful movements come from deep within our bodies and give us a profound sense of joy.

Play is by far the most under-rated and frequently-ignored element in human physical education today. We are so busy doing grim, technically-advanced warrior workouts that we have lost sight of the fundamentals, including those simple movements that give us pleasure. Fitness professionals tell us about things like strength, endurance and flexibility, but rarely do they mention the merits of simple pleasure in movement. As you will see, play is not only pleasurable, it offers concrete, tangible fitness results that rival anything that you can achieve through labor.

Sadly, we desperately need remedial education in play. For much of our young lives, big, powerful adults have pestered us to get serious and above all, grow up. Reluctantly, most of us mastered this directive, but many of us went too far and now we need instruction in the opposite direction. Giving ourselves permission to play and enjoy life is a good place to start, but we can do even better. We can say not only that play is permissible, but that it is vital, not only for the health of our individual bodies, but also for our communities and our culture as a whole. Play is essential and it's about time that we remembered how to do it. It's time to grow down.

panorama

As you will see, this book takes an ambitious, broad-ranging look at human physical conditioning. It is not a book of fitness tips that will get results in "just minutes a day." It will not reveal the secret training methods used by movie stars, Navy Seals, Green Berets, Ninja warriors or Hollywood stunt men. It will not tell you how to melt fat, banish your belly or lose your gut. It will not chisel your abs, sculpt your thighs, build massive arms or give you buns of steel. It will not make you look like a supermodel or improve your sexual performance. This is not a quick-fix method, nor is it a promotion for nutritional supplements or exercise products. This book is not a medical guide or a fitness prescription; it will not "turn back the clock," make you young again or prevent you from dying. And above all, this is not a book for Dummies, Idiots or Morons.

Rather, this book is for intelligent people who want to enjoy their bodies and expand their understanding of what it means to be physically functional and fully alive. It is a powerfully comprehensive way of thinking about the human body and performance. This book won't answer all your questions about fitness, exercise or health, but it will offer you a powerful orientation that will give meaning to your exercise and stimulate your physical creativity.

This book is different from other "body" books because it provides a broad theoretical foundation and meaningful context for fitness and exercise. It offers a synthesis of material from widely divergent disciplines. I will take you on a journey across the fields of evolution, anthropology, medicine, physiology and modern athletic training. By the time you finish this book, you will view your exercise and training practices as part of a much larger whole.

My presentation will come in six parts. In the first section, we'll look at the distressing state of the modern human body and speculate on the forces that brought us to this point. We'll look at popular fitness paradigms and ask whether or not they are actually making us any healthier or happier.

Then we'll start back at the beginning and design a program from scratch. First we'll explore our evolutionary history and speculate on what it means for modern-day health and fitness. We'll look at the characteristics of our ancestral environment and ponder the athletic feats of our ancestors. We'll evaluate some of our modern exercises and test their relevance to the history of the human body.

Next we'll look at practical, functional considerations of physical training. We'll look at the foundational concepts of exercise and explore ways to make them relevant to real-life challenges that you have to face each day. The idea is to keep exercise simple, practical and effective.

Then we'll make some mischief. Play is not only enjoyable, it is fundamental to a life of sustainable, vigorous movement. We'll look at the way that play motivates and delights us, and we'll examine a few select fitness games.

Finally, we'll wrap up the whole package and talk about ways to integrate primal perspectives, functional orientations and play into our daily lives. Fitness does not take place in isolation. To achieve success, we also need life skills and orientations that will bring movement into our daily experience. I'll share some ideas for bringing movement into your life in a way that feels natural, satisfying and meaningful.

warning

At this point in the presentation, the typical fitness book sternly warns the reader to "consult a physician before beginning an exercise program." Publishers and editors consider this to be sound, responsible medical advice, but in the context of what we now know about human evolution, we can see that this counsel is entirely backwards. This ominous warning suggests that physical stasis is the norm for the human body and that movement is the hazardous exception. It implies that the safest place for the human body is on the couch and suggests that if you actually plan on leaving the couch, you'd better talk to your doctor first. This strikes fear into the minds of many would-be exercisers and keeps them suspended in a state of inactivity and impending disease. In a very real sense, this warning is part of our problem.

The irony here is that doctors, biologists and anthropologists now know that this standard issue, boilerplate warning is completely outdated and reflects the precise opposite of the truth. The human body evolved in an environment of regular physical activity. The animal body thrives on movement; the grassland is the norm, the couch is the exception. In their landmark book *The Paleolithic Prescription,* authors Eaton, Shostak and Konner put it this way: "Viewed through the perspective of evolutionary time, sedentary existence, possible for great numbers of people only during the last century, represents a transient, unnatural aberration."

Acting together, several forces have rendered us less active and tricked us into believing that movement is something inherently hazardous. Agriculture was the first step towards a sedentary life. Farming is certainly hard work, but it also anchored us to a single location and took us out of our nomadic, hunting and gathering lifestyles. For the first time in history, human beings made their living, not by walking from place to place in search of food, but by staying put.

Not long afterwards, a rapid series of technological innovations made personal locomotion and physical labor increasingly optional. The internal combustion engine made it possible to travel great distances without walking and mechanical devices began to do our lifting for us. Suddenly, the cultural norm became inactivity. The typical human lifestyle became stationary and sedentary.

Over the course of a few short decades, this condition has come to be considered normal, even though–in the context of human evolution and animal biology–it is a radical, unhealthy departure. Today, many people see physical movement simply as another menu option that a person might choose, much like a hobby, something not appreciably different from computer gaming or wine tasting. Yes, a person could, if he or she desired, begin an exercise program, but since this is out of the ordinary, caution is advised.

We have even gone so far as to create a specialized branch of medicine directed specifically towards active people: sports medicine. The implication here is that, because they are different, athletes need their own independent brand of medical care. But active people are not different; they are normal human beings with normal medical needs. If we are going to create a specialized branch of medicine, it ought to be designed for that segment of the population that deviates from the evolutionary norm. In other words, instead of sports medicine, we ought to be developing a specialty practice called *sedentary medicine*.

This takes us to the situation we see today. In a perverse reversal of our evolutionary origins, we are now advised to "consult a physician before beginning an exercise program." The underlying assumption is that physical activity is some kind of alien state, something we are not really suited for. This, of course, is preposterous; our primal ancestors would laugh their heads off if we gave them such advice.

All of the body's systems–circulatory, digestive, immune, pulmonary and nervous–perform best in a dynamic environment. Regular movement is so absolutely central to our existence, so crucial to the quality of our lives, that we can properly say that physical inactivity is itself a disease, even in the absence of unpleasant symptoms.

Yes, there are risks that come with some kinds of movement and we surely can cross the reversal point from benefit into injury. Yes, if you've been on the couch for a couple of decades, a sudden plunge into exercise could be medically risky. But by comparison, the more substantial risk comes with stasis. In other words, if you exercise, you *might* hurt yourself. You might strain your heart or inflame the ligaments in your knees. You might twist you ankle or fall off your bike. But if you don't exercise, you will almost certainly suffer early physical degeneration and illness; your heart will become flaccid, your muscles will begin to atrophy and your nervous system will go dormant.

Thus, the warning ought to read "Before beginning a program of physical *inactivity*, consult your physician." In fact, if you're planning a lifetime of sustained sloth, you'd better get regular checkups and make sure your medical insurance is all paid up; you're probably going to need it.

The state of the body

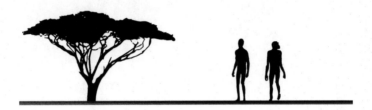

Good news, bad news

As we look at the people around us, we see an astonishing array of diverse forms and capabilities. If you're interested in bodies, you've probably found yourself wondering about the condition of your own body and the people around you. As it turns out, it's a very mixed bag.

First, the good news. Thanks to advances in scientific medicine and public health, we're living longer than ever before; the lifespan of the average North American now stands at about 80 years. We know how to prevent and cure many infectious diseases, although the edge we have enjoyed over the last few decades seems to be slipping away. We're becoming extremely adept at surgical treatments, including spectacular organ transplants and joint replacements. Modern pharmaceuticals now give us ever-finer control over our physiology, while stem cell research and biotechnology promise incredible new cures for some of our most devastating diseases. And, in one of the least appreciated developments in medical history, we have learned how to conduct effective double-blind studies and clinical trials. By bringing placebo effects to light, these methods give us authentic knowledge about what works and what doesn't. With these kinds of advances, the outlook for physical health looks promising.

Unfortunately, there's also a long list of bad news to contend with. Let's begin with the obvious. To put it bluntly, the majority of us are overweight and out of shape. We're fatter than ever before in human history. Recent studies suggest that some 60% of Americans are overweight.

We have ample evidence to document this trend, but one example is particularly stark: In January, 2003, the Federal Aviation Administration began a review process to increase the standard weight calculation for air passengers. This move came in response to the crash of a twin-engine turboprop in North Carolina earlier in the year. Investigators suspect that the cause of the crash may have been the sheer bulk of the passengers.

Even more disturbing, our kids are following our example. Never before in history have so many children been so obese. This is a genuine epidemic; the trend not only afflicts North Americans and Europeans, it is now beginning to show up in pockets all around the planet, including Asia and parts of Africa.

Not only are we overweight, we're suffering from a wide range of diseases that, in many cases, could be easily prevented with regular movement. A landmark article in the *Journal of Applied Physiology* made this point crystal clear. As lead researcher Frank Booth wrote:

> ...a strong association exists between the increase in physical inactivity and the emergence of modern chronic diseases in 20th century industrialized societies. Approximately 250,000 deaths per year in the United States are premature due to physical inactivity. Epidemiological data have established that physical inactivity increases the incidence of at least 17 unhealthy conditions, almost all of which are chronic diseases or considered risk factors for chronic diseases.

According to this review, physical inactivity is costing the American health care system nearly $1 trillion. Some epidemiologists are now suggesting that a sedentary lifestyle is as much a risk factor for disease as is smoking. It's no wonder that, in its March 2000 review of Booth's article, *Sports Medicine Digest* declared that "Americans are entwined in a fatal embrace with their couches."

In 1996, the Surgeon General released a landmark report detailing the physical condition of modern Americans. Among the findings:

> More than 60 % of American adults are not regularly physically active. In fact, 25% of Americans are not active at all...Nearly half of American

youths 12-21 years of age are not vigorously active on a regular basis. Moreover, physical activity
declines dramatically during adolescence…

Given that the relationship between activity and
several diseases is likely to be causal, it follows
that a large number of Americans unnecessarily
become ill or die each year because of an inactive
way of life. Published estimates of the number of
lives lost in a year because of inactivity have ranged
from 200,000 for inactivity alone to 300,000 for
inactivity and poor diet combined.

In a related government finding, a National Institutes of Health
Statement on Physical Activity and Cardiovascular Health identi-
fied physical inactivity as a major public health problem in the
United States.

The severity of our condition is highlighted by the recent up-
surge in Type 2 or "adult-onset" diabetes. A few decades ago, this
condition only appeared in older patients, but now, physicians are
beginning to see younger and younger patients presenting with the
condition. This now stands as a serious threat to an entire generation
of young people. In fact, some observers have speculated that today's
young people may be part of the first generation in modern times
not to outlive their parents.

functional deficiencies

That's only the beginning. Not only are we fat, needlessly sick
and chronically inactive, many of us are functionally deficient. We
can't do as much with our bodies as our recent ancestors; we can't
lift as much, walk as far or work as hard. Paleoanthropologists have
examined fossil bones and observed that the points of muscular
attachment in ancient humans were much more massive than in
modern individuals; these findings suggest a high level of raw physical strength. It is true that today's professional athletes continue to
set records and amaze us with incredible performances, but these

feats are the work of a tiny fraction of our population; the rest of us are performing at a level far below our capability.

The functional deficiencies of modern humans are not obvious to most of us because they are heavily masked by modern locomotive technologies. Cars, buses and airplanes take us where we want to go, almost on demand. Since physical challenges are now relatively rare, we just don't see how poor most peoples' condition really is. Unless you are actively involved in assessing, training or treating the physical body, you are unlikely to notice the condition. Nevertheless, we are truly in poor shape; if called upon to join the ranks of our hunting and gathering ancestors, most of us would fall behind and perish in short order.

sensory-motor amnesia

One way to describe our condition is to say that many of are afflicted by a condition known as "sensory-motor amnesia." This is not some esoteric nervous system pathology. Rather, it is a simple and highly preventable disorder. Through consistent and prolonged disuse, the human nervous system forgets how to organize and direct physical movement; we don't use it, so we lose it. In sensory-motor amnesia, the nervous system circuits that detect body position and control movement gradually go dormant. Physical sensitivity to motion atrophies and our ability to direct powerful and graceful contractions fades as well.

This is an epidemic physical condition, just as real as heart disease or osteoporosis. The reason we don't hear more about it is that, once again, it's presence is heavily masked by our transportation technologies. Just about any minimally fit person can manage to drive a car for example, so we don't notice their lack of physical capability until it becomes truly extreme. But if we were forced out of our cars and onto the open grassland of our origins, individuals with sensory-motor amnesia would become instantly obvious (to us and to predators).

body loathing

Conspicuously, we also have an epidemic of anxiety about our bodies, a nagging sense of unease that haunts many of us around the clock. Modern people do not celebrate their bodies; indeed, many of us can scarcely tolerate them. We relate to our bodies as if they were treacherous aliens, ever ready to sabotage our life experience with saggy flesh and distorted appearance. This obsession is on regular display at every news stand, where magazine covers amplify our bodily discontent into full-blown obsessions.

Our physical discontent is revealed by the fact that for today's exerciser, the most common driving motivation is not joy but fear. We don't go towards physical pleasure, invigorating movement or simple fun, we flee from sagging flesh, bulging bellies, coronary artery disease and social rejection. We don't exercise because we enjoy movement or the things that we can do when we're fit, we exercise because we hate our bodies and because exercise is the only thing that offers a realistic chance for improvement. Clearly, this kind motivation tends to be unsustainable. Who wants to participate in an exercise program whose only promise is temporary relief from the inevitable disfigurement that comes with age?

Incredibly, our obsession with thinness even afflicts those who are already fit and healthy. One researcher polled instructors at a fitness convention, using questionnaires on nutrition, figure rating and exercise activity. Presented at the American College of Sports Medicine annual meeting in 1999, the report concluded that "Women fitness instructors have a similar level of body dissatisfaction as college women and women athletes such as gymnasts, weight lifters, and marathon runners...Body dissatisfaction was independent of physical characteristics such as percent body fat or body mass index." And in *Cheers and Tears*, author Shane Murphy cites a study indicating that nearly 75% of female collegiate athletes believe that they are overweight. In other words, even thin people are distressed about their appearance.

Experts now point to the growing number of young children, especially girls, who fret about body image. In extreme but increasingly common cases, they are being treated for eating disorders. Dr. Ira Sacker, director of the eating disorder clinic at Brookdale University Hospital in Brooklyn and co-author of the book *Dying To Be Thin*, sees a trend. "These aren't isolated cases anymore," says Sacker. Studies reported in 2001 found that children as young as age 5 in Australia and Hong Kong wanted to be thinner, echoing similar U.S. findings.

It's not just women and girls who are plagued with anxiety about the shape and appearance of their bodies. Men have also gotten into the act with their own body-beautiful magazines and an affliction known as "muscle dysmorphia." This condition might be described as the flip side of anorexia; clinically, it is described as "a preoccupation with an imagined defect in appearance," especially the belief that they appear "small and weak" to those around them. Bodybuilders in particular suffer from this condition, many of whom studiously avoid exposing their bodies in public, except when in peak condition.

depression

There's more bad news, this time on the psychological front. Depression has risen dramatically over the last several decades. Reporting in 1992 and 1996 in the *Journal of the American Medical Association*, epidemiologist Myrna Weissman and colleagues found that more Americans are becoming depressed and that the severity of depression is also rising. Each generation of the 20th century has suffered more depression than the previous one; since WWII, the rate of depression has more than doubled. Not surprisingly, the use of anti-depressive medications has also skyrocketed.

The cause for this rise in depression is no doubt complex and it would be a mistake to pin the blame on any single cause. Nevertheless, we can't ignore the obvious fact that this rise in depression coincides neatly with the drastic decline in movement that we've experienced over the last one hundred years. Correlation does not mean causation, but this one is highly suggestive; take any animal, restrict its normal movement to a small fraction of its biological norm and you're bound to see changes in its brain chemistry, disposition and outlook.

overworked, underplayed

Because of our inactive lifestyles, we are losing contact with our bodies and the joy that comes with movement. A culture of workaholics, we work long hours and then, if we've got the time, we do workouts. Today's kids are booked up months in advance and have little time for spontaneous play. Impromptu after-school play sessions have all but disappeared. It scarcely comes as a surprise then, if children don't experience play when they're young, they aren't going to be playing when they get older. Many of today's children are completely unaware of the pleasure of vigorous activity. As professional sports has risen to prominence, play has now been largely replaced by spectating. In effect, we now pay other people to do our playing for us.

It is no exaggeration to say that, for individuals and for our culture as a whole, the disappearance of play is a genuine cause for alarm. We could even describe this condition in the context of public health. Even if we were to ignore the consequences of long-term sedentary living, we can say that this reduced level of physical play is itself a symptom of some deeper affliction. If field biologists were to visit our planet from another galaxy, they would surely take note of this one species that exhibits a reduced interest in play, not only compared to its historical average, but also in comparison to other similar species.

the worst is yet to come

Bad as it is, the condition of our bodies will continue to deteriorate over the coming years and decades. As our population ages, the vast number of people who are currently sedentary will begin to show up in increasing numbers in hospitals and clinics, looking for treatment. The bill for inactive living will come due in the form of even greater claims for heart disease, diabetes, hypertension, back pain and other inactivity-related diseases.

William Novelli, CEO for the American Association of Retired Persons, points to the year 2011 as a crucial pivot point for health care services. In that year, the first wave of baby-boomers will turn 65, which will put extreme pressure on our social structures, especially medical care. Because of our poor fitness, physicians and hospitals will become increasingly preoccupied with treating highly preventable disorders and medical resources will be drawn away from vital research. An already stressed medical delivery system will be pushed to the limit. Things are going to get ugly.

the magnitude of the loss

The loss of physical experience, pleasure and health that we see in today's world is not simply an unpleasant side-effect of modern living or a public-policy problem that needs to be managed; it is a genuine human tragedy. In magnitude, it is not at all unlike losing our art, our music or our literature. If a terrorist burned down a great museum, we would be aghast at the loss of an invaluable cultural gem. If an earthquake swallowed up a great symphony hall, we would lament the loss of great music. If our libraries were closed because of budget cuts, we would be furious.

But in a sense, losing contact with our bodies is an even greater catastrophe than any loss of culture. After all, our physical heritage is far, far deeper than any cultural invention. The body is our bridge to human history and to the rest of the natural world. Without a vibrant, functional body, how are we to relate to the rest of the biosphere? Primal peoples would be simultaneously mystified and appalled at our physical condition and our passive willingness to accept it as natural. If alien invaders had arrived on earth and imposed this physical atrophy upon us by external force, we would have presumably resisted it with every means possible.

Life in an alien environment

> Human nature is, moreover, a hodgepodge of spe-
> cial genetic adaptations to an environment largely
> vanished, the world of the Ice-Age hunter-gatherer.
>
> E.O. Wilson

When we try to solve the conundrum of our modern-day physical atrophy, we eventually come into contact with the study of human evolution and when we do, we are likely to come to some surprising and difficult realizations. Specifically, we come to understand that our bodies are adapted to an environment entirely different than the one we currently inhabit. We are, in a sense, living out of context.

Let's review how we got here. Most of us know that evolution is a slow process. We know that the transformation from arboreal primate to *Homo sapiens* took place over several million years, with the gradual accumulation of mutations that led to bipedal locomotion, big brains and the capacity for language. The thing that we keep forgetting is that biological evolution and cultural transformations have taken place on entirely different time scales. While it typically takes millions of years for a new species to evolve, human cultural transformation can take place almost overnight.

Beginning with the advent of agriculture, human technological innovation has exploded in a positive feedback cycle. In the course of a mere 50,000 years, we have gone from chipped stones to silicon chips, from stone huts to Pizza Hut. In the process, we have completely re-engineered our physical world and created, in effect, an environment within an environment. This human-constructed world is totally unlike any that we have previously inhabited in the course of our history.

The transformation from grassland living to present-day conditions has taken place with staggering abruptness. Agriculture–the pivotal development that led to civilization–was invented 10,000 years ago and not universally adopted until much more recently. But in terms of biological transformation, 10,000 years is a mere heartbeat. In biological terms, the transformation from hunter-gather vigor to modern-day atrophy has occurred overnight.

The thing that we keep forgetting is the fact that our genes, bodies and brains are identical to those of our hunting and gathering ancestors. There is no physical difference between human beings living 100,000 years ago and those living today–same bodies, same brains, same inclinations. If you were to build a time machine and travel backward 100,000 years, you would meet people–*Homo sapiens*–with bodies and dispositions fundamentally identical to your own. Obviously, you would not be able to converse with them, but they would be just as intelligent as you, perhaps more so. And in all likelihood, you wouldn't have the slightest chance of keeping up with any of them.

The shift from Paleolithic wildness (the "old stone age") to modernity has taken place in a biological instant. So rapid was the transformation, it is as if we were plucked from our native environment, carried across the galaxy on a transporter beam and dropped into a completely new world. Thus, we are cave men with beepers. We are Paleolithic hunters with cell phones. We are gatherers in SUVs. We are grassland adventurers cruising the strip malls. We are tribal animals working in board rooms, conference halls and high-rise office buildings.

Our bodies are supremely well adapted to the semi-wooded grassland and similar habitats; millions of years of natural selection made it so. In contrast, our bodies are not adapted to the world of cars, chairs, long work hours and cheap food. Our bodies have been sculpted for regular movement, not stasis. It is no exaggeration to say that we are now living in an alien environment.

If you've studied human origins, none of this will come as a surprise. Yes, today's world is different from the ancestral homeland; we realize that. What most of us fail to understand is the magnitude of the difference. That is, today's environment is radically different from our primal heritage. The modern shopping mall is to the ancestral grassland as an aquarium is to the open ocean. The movement challenges are so different that it is inevitable that we would suffer physical consequences.

When we come to appreciate the fact that we are living in an alien environment, lots of things suddenly become clear. Depression, anxiety, vague medical conditions; none of these things come as a surprise. Take a wild animal, pull it out of it's natural habitat, drop it into a new world with a completely novel set of physical challenges and you're bound to see a whole host of inappropriate behaviors, compensations and consequences. When your body is out of context, things just don't work right.

features of our alien environment

Today's alien environment is different from our ancestral home in several key respects. Most conspicuous is the stasis that is imposed upon our bodies by chairs, couches and cars. Some of this stasis is voluntary of course, but a lot of it is mandatory; if you want to get anywhere in today's world, you're going to have to sit still for long periods, like it or not.

Even when we do get the opportunity for movement, the quality of motion that we experience is fundamentally alien. Our ancestral habitat presented us with highly diverse terrain challenges that included dirt, sand, rocks, hills and swamps. In contrast, the terrain of today's human-built environment is extremely homogeneous. Pavement is smooth, concrete is level, floors are monotonous. Modern humans can get by with a single gait pattern, regardless of where we go. One gait, one walk, one neuromuscular pattern of movement.

Unfortunately, the monotonous terrain of the modern world produces a dumb, insensitive gait pattern and slow, injury-prone legs. Imperfections in our anatomical structure are stressed in exactly the same fashion with every step. In contrast, if you're walking on diverse terrain, you'll give those imperfections periodic rests; diverse terrain is actually far easier on the body than monotonous surfaces. In a sense, mountains are easier than treadmills.

Our modern, alien environment also leads to a general reduction in the quantity of human movement. With the exception of professional athletes and working laborers, we can accurately describe our modern population as "hypokinetic." That is, we move less frequently and with less intensity than we need to for optimal health. A sure indicator of this trend is the fact that we have essentially given up the primary movement pattern of our species, walking. A researcher at University of California reportedly calculated that the average American walks less than 75 miles per year–about 1.4 miles per week, a paltry 350 yards per day.

Compare this with the lives of our primal ancestors. If we take a conservative guess and say that the average hominid or ancient human walked a couple of miles per day (William Leonard, professor of anthropology at Northwestern University, has calculated that modern hunter-gatherers put in six to eight miles per day), we see that we are now walking significantly less than 10% of the historical average for our species. This is a radical, drastic change in a fundamental behavior. If we were to take any other animal species and restrict its normal level of movement by 90%, it's a sure bet that we'd see some serious health consequences.

In terms of the actual volume of movement, modern society actually has a great deal in common with prison populations. Correctional facilities vary widely in how much exercise is permitted for inmates, but in general, the whole idea of prison is to restrict movement. Nevertheless, some prisoners do take advantage of institutional exercise facilities and manage to maintain good fitness levels. The tragic irony is that many of today's incarcerated felons actually get more exercise than the typical free man or woman. In other words, many of today's moderns might actually become fitter and healthier if they were serving time.

Another way to describe our alien environment is to say that it tends to produce chronic stress deficiencies. This may sound surprising, given our current mania for stress reduction programs and therapies. Nevertheless, stress–especially physical stress–is a vital part of health and fitness.

The tissues of our musculoskeletal system–our muscles, tendons, ligaments and bones–cannot thrive in a state of suspended animation; they depend on gravitational, resistive and kinetic loads to maintain their integrity and health. When muscle tissue is challenged, it responds with growth and increased neural drive; it learns to generate stronger contractions. When connective tissue fibers are challenged with repeated contractions, they supercompensate by growing thicker at crucial junctions. When bones are loaded repeatedly, they increase their mineral density along the axes of greatest force. In this, stress is not the enemy at all; in fact, it is the primary somatic teacher that tells us where to grow, what to reinforce and how to heal.

Without some sort of physical challenge, all tissues of the musculoskeletal system become weak and injury prone. In this sense, we can accurately speak of gravitational, kinetic and resistive stresses, not as injury-promoting forces, but as nourishment. Our tissues need stress and loading just as much as they need optimal amounts of proteins, fats and carbohydrates; in this sense, it is no exaggeration to say that physical stress is food.

Researchers have studied the effects of prolonged inactivity by placing volunteers in bed for up to three weeks after a control period in which baseline measurements were taken. According to the Surgeon General's report, "The resulting detrimental changes in physiological function and performance are similar to those resulting from reduced gravitational forces during space flight." These include profound decrements in cardiorespiratory function, glucose intolerance/insulin resistance, negative nitrogen balance (reflecting loss of muscle protein), negative calcium balance (reflecting loss of bone mass) and progressive decrement in skeletal muscle mass (atrophy).

Science fiction buffs like to imagine what human life would be like if we were living in space, cruising the solar system or rocketing to distant galaxies. This sounds like grand speculation, a fantasy life in some distant future. But in one sense at least, such a life is already upon us. In terms of movement demands and physical challenges, we are, for all practical purposes, living in space right now. In fact, there are astronauts on the space shuttle who get more exercise than the average American.

We now live in a world where gravitational, kinetic and resistive stresses are largely optional. Automobiles and aircraft take us where we want to go and hydraulic machines lift the things we need.

Many of us sit for hours at a time each day and experience virtually no musculoskeletal challenge whatsoever. So, while our bodies are bulging with caloric overload, they are simultaneously starving for kinetic, gravitational and resistive nourishment; a great percentage of the disabilities that we suffer can be properly be called underuse injuries. What we need is physical stress and lots of it.

inappropriate impulses

Unfortunately, our innate physical instincts don't always serve us well in this new, alien world. Take our inclination towards physical rest and relaxation for example. Throughout human history, vigorous and frequent physical movement has been the compulsory norm. Our ancestors were motivated by natural forces including bad weather, wildfires, food scarcity, insects, predation and possible aggression from other tribes. The environment forced us to move; in many cases, movement was mandatory. Living in these kinds of conditions, it simply made good sense to rest whenever possible. If hunger, heat and carnivores are chasing you across the landscape, you'll take any opportunity to lounge in the shade.

If you think of animals living in wild settings, it becomes obvious that slothful behaviors are an asset; in evolutionary terms, it pays to be lazy. In fact, any organism that engages in movement beyond environmental and reproductive necessity is taking an unnecessary risk. To put it another way, any creature that conserves physical resources is in a far better position to endure the inevitable physical challenges that are bound to appear. In a sense, the evolutionary rewards go, not to the greatest achievers, but to the slackers who recline most effectively.

At this point, we come face to face with a surprising distinction. That is, while play and regular vigorous movement is the norm for hominids and humans, and is therefore natural, exercise is something else altogether. While vigorous movement is completely natural, this thing we call "exercise"–optional, non-essential, structured movement–is a highly unnatural act. For the same reason, sport and athletics must also be considered "unnatural."

For the last few decades, we have been inundated with exercise and fitness information that, for the most part, has only served to make people feel guilty. Everyone from Jane Fonda to the Surgeon General has pleaded with us to get us off the couch, and yet most of us find some excuse to recline. Puritanical trainers call this a character flaw, but I call it a natural by-product of evolution. We are bums because our grandfather hominids were bums and because it worked to be a bum. We are horribly out of shape for one simple reason: the right thing feels wrong and the wrong thing feels right.

Today, fossil fuels do most of our labor for us and personal locomotion has become largely optional. In this context, our inclination towards sloth is no longer so adaptive. In fact, it is downright dangerous. It dupes us into compulsive reclining, and since we aren't compelled to run towards or away from anything, our bodies begin to degenerate. What was once an asset is now a liability.

For animals in the wild, the default physical programming says "Rest now because you never know when the next challenge might be coming. When in doubt, rest." There is no ambiguity here. Even the casual observer of the natural world can see that wild animals do not "work out." Play, hunt or flee, yes, but exercise—never. In the entire history of biology and zoology, we have yet to observe any non-human animal doing anything remotely resembling a modern human "workout," and yet they remain generally healthy. If primates actually needed workouts for health, Jane Goodall would have reported that the chimps at Gombe were pumping rocks and running laps around the forest. In fact, she reported no such thing.

So now we're facing a difficult conundrum. Our bodies are programmed to rest whenever possible, but the movement demands that we have lived with for millions of years have disappeared. And now our trainers, coaches and physicians are telling us to get moving. It's no wonder that we ignore them.

The magnitude of this challenge is immense. We can spin it any way we like, but there is just no getting around the fact that, like our ancestors, we are lazy hominids who like to lie in the shade and eat the best that the grassland has to offer. Give me a barbecue, a six-pack and a good playoff series on TV and I'm a happy guy.

Our problems with health and fitness are not simply those of failure to exercise or failure to eat the right foods. Our problems are of an entirely different order. The challenge that we are facing is unprecedented in human history. We don't know how to live in this alien world and for the most part, no one is teaching us.

In degree and in kind, promoting exercise is not unlike trying to promote sexual abstinence or rigid dietary restriction; these things simply go against the evolutionary grain and our bodies revolt. In this way, today's health and fitness challenge takes an interesting twist. It's not a matter of numbers, body fat percentages or oxygen uptake. Rather, the primary objective in health and fitness is figuring out how to live in an alien world.

The cult of cosmetics

Just as our bodies do not exist in isolation, our current state of physical atrophy does not exist in isolation either. Our condition is the result of our choices, behaviors and orientations, all of which are shaped by our culture. Thus, we can't really hope to get ourselves back into shape unless we take our culture into account.

Unfortunately, our ideas about fitness, health, exercise and movement are now dominated by a cosmetic paradigm that dictates how we think about our bodies. The exercises we do, the goals that we aspire to, the training practices we employ, are consistently dominated by appearance. Our bodies, it seems, are ruled by magazine covers.

It's no secret that we live in a culture that places immense value on bodily appearance. Our fashion, cosmetics and publishing industries capitalize on the insecurities of normal-looking people and feed these insecurities with a constant parade of exceptional images. This in turn leads directly to our maniacal obsession with weight loss. We now spend more than thirty billion dollars per year in an effort to shed unwanted pounds. Some surveys now suggest that nine out of ten women feel bad about some aspect of their bodies. This condition is so pervasive and all-consuming that many people now believe that exercise exists for no other purpose than losing weight.

In the fitness world, appearance now overshadows almost every other consideration, including the ability to move effectively and joyously. We see dozens of publications that promote, brazenly or covertly, the skinny and youthful ideal. Even runner's magazines, once an advocate functional performance, are now promoting the weight loss angle.

The extent of our obsession is staggering. In 2002, the New York-based Council on Size and Weight Discrimination reported that young American women are more afraid of being overweight than they are of nuclear war or cancer. According to a 1991 study published in the *International Journal of Eating Disorders*, 42% of female students between grades 1 and 3 say they want to be thinner, and 51% of nine and 10 year-olds feel better about themselves if they're on a diet. A range of horrifying "pro-anorexia" websites now promote eating disorders as "a lifestyle choice."

how this affects our movement patterns

The tyranny of appearance affects our lives in many ways. Not only does it distort our self-esteem and our relationships with one another, it also changes the way that we exercise. It takes us away from play and joyous movement and drives us towards highly repetitive movement, shaping, toning and anabolic building programs. No longer do we practice movement as something to be relished for its inherent pleasure, we tolerate it as a monotonous means to a cosmetic end.

Our cosmetic orientation also has a strong influence on the way that we select movements. When our interest is in play, we seek out vigorous, diverse and dynamic movements that bounce and swing on the edge of instability. We look for moves that are slightly unpredictable in their outcome, moves that entail a certain degree of risk. We'll wrestle, play with a ball, skip across the field and do hop scotch.

When our interest is appearance on the other hand, we look for maximum calorie burning and anabolic, muscle-building effects. In particular, we look for repetitious movements that can be sustained for a really long time; this leads us to long-distance running, stationary bikes, treadmills and stairclimbers. These movements are inherently boring and thus we need additional motivation and distraction provided by televisions and loud music. And, if our interest is muscle building, we'll look to ways to drive our muscles to failure in a small set of movement types, a repertoire that also becomes monotonous, not to mention biomechanically dysfunctional. Neither of these movement types are even remotely playful.

To make matters worse, our cosmetic orientation also shifts our attention away from whole body performance and towards one or two tissue types. The dedicated weight loss scholar knows everything about adipose tissue for example, just as the dedicated bodybuilder knows everything about muscle tissue. But both of these orientations distract us from the ultimate tissue that we really need to address, the nervous system. The nervous system controls everything that happens in the body and is ultimately responsible for the totality of our performance—our strength, endurance, flexibility, agility, balance, speed, grace and injury resistance. And, because it directs hormone concentrations and metabolism, it also has a profound effect on adipose tissue and muscle mass, in other words, our appearance. If we only pay attention to one or two tissue types, it is inevitable that we will miss the bigger physiological picture.

The limitations of our cosmetic orientation become obvious when we apply it to other systems of the body. How, for example, would you respond if the magazine cover promised you "10 days to a lean and sexy liver"? What if a personal trainer told you that he'd "slim down your respiratory system?" Hopefully, you would say that these things are crazy. After all, what we want in a liver is an organ that can metabolize chemicals efficiently; in other words, we want a liver that is functional. What we want in a respiratory system are tissues that can absorb large quantities of oxygen and deliver it to the circulatory system. The same reasoning goes for all the other systems of the body; a good system is one that works.

So why then do so many of us insist on using an entirely different standard to evaluate the musculoskeletal system? What we really want in a musculoskeletal system are tissues that can effectively move us from place to place with grace, ease and power. Why do we say that all the other systems of the body must work well, but the muscles have only to look good? Even worse, why do we seem to disregard function entirely, favoring the thin and inept over the stout and functional? Or the massively overbuilt over the graceful and competent? This is a ridiculous perversion of the human body.

Sure, appearance is important. Everyone wants to look good. We care about how other people respond to our body's appearance. But the musculoskeletal system does not exist to make us look good; it exists for locomotion. It exists to move our bodies from place to place—originally on the grasslands of East Africa and later on an epic migration across the globe. As with all animals, the function of the muscular system it to produce movement; appearance is secondary. If we rank appearance over function, training errors and eventual injury are inevitable.

it's not healthy

Unfortunately, our fixation on appearance has also led us to some serious misunderstandings about the ways that appearance relates to health. We've all heard warnings about the dire health effects of obesity for example, and many of us have come to the conclusion that our cosmetic and health ideals are identical. We have come to believe that being skinny not only makes us attractive, it also keeps us out of the hospital. In fact, the story is far more complicated.

In 1984, Covert Bailey wrote a book called *Fit or Fat?* implying, it would seem, that we are either one or the other. This suggestion tapped into a strong, but highly flawed assumption in modern culture, a two-valued approach to body appearance that says you're either gorgeous or fat.

As a marketing move, Bailey's title was perfect, but as an accurate description of human bodies, it was misleading. In fact, the correlation between body fat percentage and physical functionality is relatively weak. That is, it is entirely possible to be "fit *and* fat" or, at the other end of the spectrum, "skinny *and* physically dysfunctional."

Many of today's exercisers believe that the correlation between general health and body fat is tight, even absolute. We believe that thin is healthy and fat is unhealthy. If we can just stay thin, we'll be healthy and we'll be attractive too. Of course, at the extreme of obesity, being fat is clearly unhealthy. No one can doubt that being 30% over your normal weight puts you at risk for heart disease and diabetes. If you're that fat, you're probably not fit either.

But things just are not that simple. As with every human characteristic, there is a wide variation in "normal." To say that there is an ideal weight or body fat percentage is akin to saying that there is an ideal human height. But we know that there is a huge range in normal for many physical characteristics—blood pressure, triglycerides, hormone levels, neurotransmitters—all of these quantities span a range in human bodies. Thus, the amount of adipose tissue you happen to be carrying around is unlikely to have a direct effect on your physical functionality or your health, except in extreme cases.

Medical scientists are now bringing the true nature of the fit-fat relationship to light. The April 2000 issue of *Sports Medicine Digest* suggested that, in terms of longevity, "it's better to be fit than thin." Citing findings from the Cooper Center for Aerobics Research, they reported that, in terms of general health as measured in death rates, being fit is far more important than being thin. For out-of-shape men, obesity was clearly associated with higher death rates, but among those who were in shape, body fat percentage was unrelated to mortality. In fact, men who are fit and fat have a death rate about one half that of unfit men in the normal weight range. In other words, fit-fat beats unfit-thin; if you're capable of sustained physical movement, it doesn't matter much if you're carrying around a few extra pounds. Or to put it another way, you can increase your fitness and reduce your life-threatening health risks independently of weight loss.

Steven Blair, director of research at the Cooper Institute for Aerobics Research in Dallas has suggested that previous studies linking obesity and death from heart disease and other major killers have missed the important influence of exercise. "There is a misdirected obsession with weight and weight loss," he said. "The focus is all wrong, it's fitness that is the key."

This all makes perfect sense in terms of evolution. Imagine a troop of baboons or a tribe of chimps foraging their way across some primeval grassland. Food supplies are naturally variable and inconsistent; animals are bound to experience periods of scarcity with occasional times of abundance. Suppose these animals have been living lean for awhile, but suddenly encounter a rich, fertile valley, full of ripe fruit and other delectables. Obviously, they're going to eat as much as they want and stay as long as they like. And, they're going to eat more than they really need at that moment, so their bodies are going to store the excess calories as glycogen and fat. But there is no reason to suppose that this would have a negative health consequence; in fact, the ability to store excess calories as fat is a very healthy thing indeed. After a few weeks, you'll have a bunch of healthy primates who just happen to be packing more adipose tissue than they did before. In fact, if you're living in an unpredictable, wild environment, being fit *and* fat is an ideal combination.

Of course, in today's world, individuals who are both fit and fat—the capable corpulent—are relatively rare. If you start exercising with intensity and regularity, you'll probably lose some weight; your form will follow function. And, if you want to maximize your longevity, recent research suggests that the ideal combination is to be both fit and slender. Nevertheless, the whole thing begins with fitness. No matter how much you weigh, regular movement is essential.

before and after

The folly of the cosmetic paradigm is vividly illustrated in the notorious "before and after" photo spreads we see in so many health and fitness publications. You've seen hundreds of them. Mr. Before is chubby, sloppily dressed and unattractive to the opposite sex. Mr. After, on the other hand, is a svelte, well-dressed and confident athlete, as well as a powerful sex magnet. The same goes for Miss Before and Miss After, only more so.

By themselves, these pictures don't really tell us very much about the condition of the individuals involved, even in those cases when the photos are authentic. Consider Mr. After. He looks great to be sure, but what about his blood pressure? What about the elasticity of his coronary arteries? What about the mineral density of his bones? What about his injury-resistance and his endurance? What about the quality of his movement? What is he capable of? Is he strong enough to lift a sack of concrete into a truck? Can he hike with a backpack? How would he perform in the ancestral environment? What about the state of his nervous system? Are his neural connections any faster or more precise than before? Is his balance good? Is his body any smarter now than it was before? And, to put an even finer point on it, is he any happier? Can he do more of the things that he likes to do? These are not things that we can tell by looking at snapshots.

In fact, as a method for evaluating health and fitness, a visual assessment is useful only in the most extreme circumstances. Yes, if we look at an individual who is 5 feet tall and weighs 300 pounds, we can probably assume that his body fat percentage is too high and that his blood pressure, cardiac function and insulin responses are all in the danger zone. But that's about it. For the vast majority of people, appearance remains a poor indicator of overall health and fitness, much as the magazines would like us to believe otherwise.

We get a lesson in this every four years when we watch the Olympics. We know that virtually all of the competitors have beautiful bodies; these people look great. But it is simply not the case that the best looking bodies win all the gold medals. In fact, there are lots of beautifully sculpted bodies that don't even qualify for the competition. If appearance correlated precisely with performance, there wouldn't be any reason to have the Olympics at all; we'd just put everyone up on stage, pick out the best-looking bodies and be done with it.

The same is true throughout the sporting world. There are some really chiseled bodies in the NBA, for example, but they don't necessarily rise to the top of the scoring charts. In fact, if you've ever seen a picture of Michael Jordan with his shirt off, you'd be surprised to see that he looks stunningly, disappointingly average. His muscles are of normal size, shape and tone. (But man, what a nervous system!)

If you ever want a demonstration of the relative importance of function and cosmetics in human life, just ask someone who has suffered one or the other. Loss of cosmetic beauty is obviously undesirable, but a loss of function is catastrophic. Sportsmedicine physicians and supportive spouses are quite familiar with the laments of athletes who can no longer do their sport. But out in the real world, the lost ability to throw a curve ball is nothing. If you want a true sense of how a loss of function can affect a human life, ask someone in a wheelchair. Ask someone whose back hurts so much that they can't go to work or keep their house in order. Across the board, these people would trade almost any cosmetic quality to have their function back. Fat and functional is a condition that we can live with. In contrast, a loss of function is torture and must be avoided at all possible cost.

no magic pill

Because of our obsession with appearance and weight-loss, too many people misunderstand the nature and magnitude of the challenge that we face. We tend to concentrate on the obvious, thinking that our biggest physical problem is being overweight. If we could just solve that physiological puzzle–so we think–then all would be well with our bodies. Indeed, the promise lies just out there on the scientific horizon. As biochemists team up with pharmacologists, we inch ever closer to an understanding of the physiology of appetite and in turn, a magic pill that would truly make us lose weight; the magic "eat all you want" pill.

But such a pill, even if it worked as advertised, would not come close to solving our physical woes. Yes, we might be able to suppress appetite, accelerate metabolism and in turn, strip off unwanted body fat. But while it might make us look better, it wouldn't have any impact on our other inactivity-related disorders. Without increasing our level of physical activity, we would still suffer from a broad spectrum of physical consequences. In the end, we would simply be skinny, physically dysfunctional and disease-prone variants of our former selves. And while we might be close to finding a sure-fire weight-loss pill, we aren't anywhere near finding a pharmacological substitute for vigorous physical activity. This is something for which a technological solution seems not only distant, but impossible to imagine. The only way out of our conundrum is actual, authentic movement.

Appearance is good for something, to be sure. There can be no denying that in a beauty-conscious society, people are going to seek out whatever cosmetic edge they can get. When we look good, we feel better. But as a basis for creating an intelligent exercise method, appearance is a distraction. As you'll see, there are far better ways to think about human movement.

The tyranny of sport

Next to cosmetics, our other primary source of information about physical conditioning is the world of sport. When we participate in athletics or observe as fans, we come away with a set of ideas about how our bodies work and how we ought to be training them.

Obviously, sport has now become a dominating cultural preoccupation. No longer a leisure pastime or an single element in a well-rounded education, sport now delivers a constant stream of messages, both overt and covert, about the nature of our bodies and what we ought to be doing with them. It tells us how we measure up and what we ought to aspire to.

Clearly, there is value in modern athletics. Today's coaches and athletic trainers have amassed a huge body of valuable knowledge about how the body works. They are adept at improving specialized physical performance and getting more out of human bodies than anyone thought possible. By virtue of their vast, highly-concentrated experience with athletes, they know what it takes to stimulate the training response. They know how to fine tune the details of physical challenge for the best results. They know about periodization, biomechanics, over-training and under-training. Some of this knowledge is extremely valuable, not just to athletes, but to every human being on the planet. It could be particularly valuable to sedentary people who desperately need to get back into shape.

Nevertheless, this detailed knowledge is part of a sporting culture that has some profound social and health care negatives. Ironically, the institution with the greatest promise for promoting widespread health and fitness simultaneously tends to promote the precise opposite.

When faced with the problem of poor physical health in our population, many people reflexively promote athletics, suggesting that sports are the solution to our problem. But increasingly, a number of physical educators and observers are suggesting the exact opposite–that sport, far from being the solution to our physical malaise, is actually a big part of the problem.

Sport advocates are quick to tell us that athletics is an excellent means of building health and fitness. A quick look at the professionals seems to bear this out; these individuals are obviously in great condition. But if we take a broader perspective and look at the effects of sport on our population at large, we see an entirely different picture. That is, sport is failing to deliver on it's promise.

The popularity of athletics in North America is at an all-time high. We have more sports, more leagues, more franchises and more broadcasts than ever before in history. If sport was really an effective means of health and fitness promotion, we would expect to see a population of generally healthy and fit individuals. But as the Surgeon General has pointed out, our physical condition has never been worse. In fact, what we're now seeing is an inverse correlation between sport and general fitness of our population; as sport has become more popular, our level of health and fitness has actually declined.

The problem begins with children's athletic programs. Fred Engh is president of the National Alliance for Youth Sports. In his book, *Why Johnny Hates Sports*, Engh points out some disturbing facts about the state of youth sports: "Studies show that an alarming 70% of the approximately 20 million children who participate in organized out-of-school athletic programs will quit by the age of thirteen because of unpleasant sports experiences."

Upon reading these statistics, readers are likely to assume that there must be something wrong with the programs in question. But in one sense, there is nothing wrong with this picture at all. Sport–at least the way it is conducted in today's culture–is designed intentionally to weed out the vast majority of the participants. High drop-out numbers don't constitute a failure of sport, they constitute success. The problem is not that we don't do sport well; the problem is that we do it too well.

In today's youth sports environment, it's no longer enough to simply let children enjoy a game of baseball or football and let it go at that. No, we've got to get serious. We've got to model our programs after the pros. We've got to have a pre-season, a regular season and divisions and standings and stats and records and playoffs, all so that we can eliminate the weaker performers from contention.

The end result is that sport tends to polarize modern society. Through systematic competition and elimination, today's athletic culture divides our population into two groups; a handful of elite, physically gifted individuals who can make it as professionals, and everyone else, the spectators.

In turn, this pushes us towards two lifestyle extremes. On one hand, we have a small population of athletic extremists and special-ists. These people either succeed as athletic professionals or become chronic consumers of sports medicine. On the other hand we get a huge population of sedentary individuals, those who ultimately give up on the idea of exercise altogether. In sum, the system just doesn't work. As Shane Murphy put it in his book, *The Cheers and the Tears,* "As a vehicle for sponsoring mass participation in physical activity, youth sports programs are a huge failure."

sport and health

One of our biggest misconceptions about sport is that it promotes fitness and therefore good health. In fact, as it is conducted today, sport really has very little to do with promoting health. This is made abundantly clear by the rising epidemic of sports injuries at all levels of participation, professional and amateur, adults and children. As competition intensifies, training becomes more abstracted, frequent and demanding. We see longer training sessions, longer seasons, special training camps and twice-a-day workouts.

Women are now suffering an epidemic of ruptured anterior cruciate ligaments in their knees, professional football players are frequently crippled in early retirement and young gymnasts begin fighting overuse injuries even before they're out of childhood. Non-steroidal anti-inflammatory drugs are consumed like candy and competitive runners commonly joke about taking their "Vitamin I" (Ibuprophen), even in the face of evidence of its harmful effects. Add to this the rising intake of anabolic and performance-enhanc-ing supplements by professionals and high schoolers alike, driven in no small measure by the dictate that we "just do it." Make no mistake, sport is not about health; it is about achievement.

From the physical educator's point of view, competitive athletics actually teaches us some extremely bad habits about our bodies. Yes, sporting competitions can promote vitality, strength, speed and endurance–characteristics that are desirable for any body in any situation. But at the same time, they also teach athletes to train through pain and to suppress subtle symptoms that give them vital feedback about the condition of their bodies.

To succeed in today's intensely competitive sporting environment, athletes must put performance before health. As sport becomes a full-time career path, physical intelligence and good judgment take a back seat to execution. Sensible care of your body will not win you a gold medal or even a scholarship. Sports commentators praise the warrior spirit of the athlete who "plays in pain." In fact, playing in pain is quite often a sign of poor judgment.

Suppose that you're a baseball pitcher. Your team is struggling to make the playoffs and your spot on the roster is in jeopardy; give up a few more runs and you'll lose that scholarship or fat contract. But now you feel a pain in your rotator cuff when you throw your curve ball. Simple intelligence would suggest that you give up pitching for a while and allow the tissue to heal; from a physical educator's point of view, this is the smart and sustainable thing to do. But since your athletic career hinges on continued performance, you'll keep pitching. If this was an occasional incident, you could probably endure the trauma, but for most of today's athletes, this denial of physical feedback has become routine. It's no wonder that so many middle-age athletes are in chronic pain. Tragically, modern sport cripples our best performers while it eliminates everyone else.

The problems with sport are well-known to physiologists who understand how intense exercise affects the human body. Eric Widmaier is a professor of biology at Boston University. In his book *Why Geese Don't Get Obese*, he describes the effects of exercise and stress on ancient and modern humans. When exercise becomes too extreme or sustained, it begins to eat into metabolic reserves that are normally dedicated to reproduction or reserved for genuine emergencies. In elite female gymnasts and ballerinas, the demands are so intense that many participants stop having menstrual cycles, a condition known as exercise-induced amenorrhea. This delays the onset of puberty and may have long-range effects on growth and bone health. Widmaier views athletics this way: "As a physiologist, I cringe every time I see these young athletes performing on the world stage, as in the Olympics. It is a grossly abnormal situation, and one can only imagine what psychological effects it must have as well."

movement specialization

The other problem with modern sport is that it encourages a high degree of movement specialization. We reserve our highest accolades and rewards for those individuals who refine single movements or small sets of movements to the highest possible level. Conversely, we offer no rewards to individuals who achieve a balanced set of physical capabilities, people who strike a healthy balance between strength, endurance and agility. If you can throw a football or sink a three point shot consistently, we'll cheer your achievement and reward you outrageously, but if you're just generally fit and healthy, we'll ignore you entirely. But extreme movement specialization, as physical therapists are now beginning to discover, is a recipe for injury. If you take a single movement and practice it relentlessly for a few years, injury is almost inevitable.

Not only that, movement specialization has negative social consequences. Athletic specialization tends to isolate and divide physically active people from one another. Basketball specialists don't play with soccer specialists, sprinting specialists don't play with marathon runners. And of course, children sport specialists can't play with the kid next door; we have to take them all the way across town to find someone who knows how to move just like they do so they can compete.

Even pro-sport publications are beginning to recognize this trend towards specialization in modern athletics. In the fall of 2002, *Sports Illustrated* ran a four-part series on high school sports. Author Alexander Wolff noted the "marked trend towards specialization" and observed that "the win-at-all-costs priorities commonplace in college sports have seeped into grades 12, 11, 10 and below…As

coaches demand year-round proof of dedication, kids spend a greater and greater proportion of time practicing rather than playing."

arbitrary movement challenges

If our goal was to promote human health, we would design movements challenges intentionally. In contrast, most athletic games are
simply arbitrary physical inventions. With the possible exception of
some track and field events, most sports and athletic contests are
simply made-up games that have no relevance or relationship to any
larger context. This arbitrary nature of sport is revealed by the simple
fact that we can make up a new game any time we like. Just as we
made up cricket, bowling, golf and ping-pong, we could invent any
combination of movements and call it a sport. But just because we
invent a sport doesn't mean that it's relevant to human experience or
good for the human body. We can teach a dog to walk on it's hind
legs, but that is just a trick that has nothing whatsoever to do with
the creature's history, form or function; it is merely an entertaining
curiosity. In fact, many of today's sports resemble nothing so much
as a human circus acts, the hominid equivalent of teaching dogs to
walk on their hind legs.

extinguishes play

The other problem with sport is that it tends to extinguish our
sense of play, especially when practiced at today's level of intensity.
It used to be that the simple act of playing a game was enough to
satisfy our needs for movement and pleasure. Games provided some
structure and allowed us to channel our abundant energies. But in
today's sporting culture, outcome has eclipsed all other considerations, especially play. Children's leagues are nearly as competitive
as the pros; the emphasis is almost exclusively on execution, performance and winning. Thus, kids now do structured, organized
workouts, not play sessions.

The atrophy of our playful spirit becomes obvious when we look
at the spectacle of today's sidelines, not only in professional games,
but in children's sports as well. What we see is a rising tide of insults,
jeering, brawling and assaults. Some school districts have now insti-
tuted rules and workshops aimed at curbing inappropriate sideline

behavior. We're also seeing an increase in lawsuits leveled at coaches and youth athletic programs, many of them seeking redress for lost playing time, benchings and failure to advance to post-season tournaments. In today's youth sports, it's not how much fun you're having, it's whether you win or lose that counts.

As competition increases in youth sports programs, children come under mounting pressure to perform at high levels. A study by the Minnesota Amateur Sports Commission found that 45% of the children surveyed said that they had been called names, yelled at or insulted; 21% said that they had been pressured to play with an injury; 17% said that they had been hit, kicked or slapped; 8% said that they had been pressured to intentionally harm others. With experiences like these, it is no wonder that so many kids give up on games and movement.

age segregation

One of the most conspicuous features of modern sport is the way that it deepens the divide between young people and adults. Adults don't play sporting games with their children; they watch from the bleachers. This relationship sends a simple message to children–children play, adults spectate. Movement is for kids and professional athletes, grandstanding is for everyone else. If you want to start acting like a grown-up, stop playing and start spectating.

Naturally, people will say that it has to be this way, that we can't mix big adults and small children on the same football field or the same basketball floor–kids will just end up getting hurt. This is obviously the case for contact sports, but then again, there is nothing to say that we are compelled to play football, baseball and basketball. There are other ways to play that can safely include people of all ages and abilities. For example, this kind of multi-age, multi-ability training goes on in martial art schools all the time. Adult black belts play vigorous sparring games with white belts of all ages and both benefit.

We also see kind of cross-age play in rock climbing gyms, where adults and children take turns climbing problems and figuring out novel ways to do difficult moves. There are thousands of ways to integrate adults and children into the same activities; all it takes is some imagination.

extrinsic rewards

Sport takes us away from physical education in other ways as well. As youth sport becomes more organized and structured, we build more and more extrinsic rewards into the system. It's not good enough for kids to just to play games anymore; we've got to make sure that everyone gets some kind of take-home prize: T-shirts, ribbons, medals or trophies.

As these extrinsic rewards become more commonplace, they begin to obscure the original point of the endeavor and replace it with something altogether different. Just as some children now believe that the purpose of school is to "get grades" and that the purpose of work is to "get money," many young athletes now focus on the prizes, not the process. Sport is something that we now do for achievement, not for pleasure. The purpose is to "get medals."

Eventually, of course, young people are smart enough to figure out that, in the world of adult sports, the rewards only go to the truly gifted, while the vast majority of participants are simply kicked out of the system. The chance of extrinsic reward disappears, but now there's nothing left to take its place. People quit exercising, never having learned that the experience has great rewards of it's own.

the atrophy of physical education

The growth of sport and athletics in modern culture has been matched by a simultaneous atrophy of physical education programs. Ironically, the definitive statement on this condition appeared in *Sports Illustrated*, July 10, 2000:

> By devoting too many resources to organized competition and too few to broad, non-competitive fitness programs, the U.S. is producing a generation of kids beset with such health problems as non-insulin-dependent diabetes, cardiovascular disorders and osteoporosis, as well as common obesity, which has doubled among youth in the

last decade. Physical education used to be an important component of school life, but that has changed. The percentage of high school students enrolled in daily gym classes declined from 42% to 29% during the '90s, and 14% of people age 12 to 21 get no exercise at all.

Physical education has atrophied to such an extreme that it has almost ceased to be recognized as an authentic discipline; many people now assume that there is nothing more to physical education than learning the rules of baseball, football and basketball.

In actual fact, sport and physical education are two entirely different things. Sports are movement specialties that may or may not have anything to do with developing broad physical capabilities of the human body. The competitive format is designed specifically and intentionally to eliminate the majority of the participants from the process, leaving only the most proficient. If contestants become physically educated along the way, that's all fine and good, but it's really not really the point.

Sport and physical education do overlap on occasion, and it is sometimes the case that, by playing a sport, young people do become more physically adept. But when this succeeds, it is by accident, not by intention. Yes, if you play baseball long enough, you might develop a comprehensive set of physical skills such as agility, strength and endurance. But today's athletes are highly specialized and in this respect, many of them do not display high levels of physical intelligence or general ability when faced with novel physical challenges. Competition rewards specialization and rejects general movement skill.

This is something that our culture seems utterly incapable of understanding. That is, children playing baseball are not engaged in physical education; they are playing a game that just happens to be physical. Even gymnastics has been torn from its physical education roots and transformed into a ruthlessly competitive specialty that exists, not for the sake of the children involved, but for the sake of those who are entertained by watching.

Physical education, in its most classic form, was intended to teach general movement skills to meet a broad range of challenges. Ideally, it is broadly egalitarian and equally available to all students. Whereas only the very best can succeed in sport, everyone should be able to succeed in physical education.

Physical education actually could be a rich, authentic discipline, one with guts, especially if we cross-fertilized it with newly discovered knowledge about human origins. It could be a rigorous study, every bit as serious as physics, math or English. There's a whole world of fascinating study here, one that touches many other aspects of our lives. There's physics here, and chemistry, physiology and gobs of neuroscience. There's history too, and science and evolution. If we could give up our obsession with sport for awhile, we might discover that physical education can teach us a lot more than we thought.

a complete education

The classic Greek ideal held that athletic training was an important part of the total educational experience, but only a part. They accorded the body equal dignity with the mind and associated sport with philosophy, music, literature, painting and sculpture. The emphasis was on balance and harmony.

This vision persisted into the 20th century, where our great universities held physical education to be vital for the well-rounded individual. This perspective was personified by Roger Bannister, the first person to run a mile under 4 minutes. In one sense, Bannister was not an athlete at all, not in the way we understand the role today. Yes, he trained regularly and intensely, but he was an amateur and running was but a single element in his total education. "Running was only a small part of my life," he said. "I thought the ideal was the complete man, who had a career outside of sport."

After setting the record, Bannister quietly went on to become a respected physician. In contrast, modern athletics is considered an ideal in it's own right, completely divorced from any broader education—not a means to an end, but an end in itself. Education has now become a distant Plan B, an option for those who can't make it on the court or the playing field. The Greeks would be appalled.

In giving priority to sport, we fail to teach even basic elements of functional physical education. In effect, here's what we're telling our children: "We'll teach you how to throw a baseball, but we won't teach you how to lift a box of nails, move a piece of furniture or hike on a trail. We'll teach you how to set up a zone defense, but we won't teach you how to develop useful balance and strength in your legs. We'll teach you how to swim across a pool in a flash, but we won't teach you how to prevent injuries. We'll make sure that you know how to swing a golf club, but if you want to know how to keep your heart in working order, that's something you're going to have to find out on your own."

a public health problem

Most Americans believe that athletics plays a vital role in promoting health and fitness. In isolated cases this is certainly true, but for our culture as a whole, sport is now becoming a serious health negative. By relentlessly selecting only the best for participation and advancement, we leave a vast class of people to become passive spectators and life-long fans. These people become inactive and in many cases, go on to become ill with hypokinetic disorders such as heart disease and diabetes, which in turn puts tremendous pressure on our health care system. In this sense, it is only a slight exaggeration to say that sport–as it is now conducted–constitutes a significant public health problem. To the extent that sports drives thousands of people out of participation each year, sport contributes strongly to our general pattern of inactivity and the health problems that go with it.

Starting from scratch

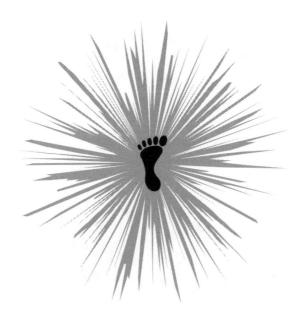

A new enlightenment

Clearly, our current paradigms for health and physical education just aren't working. For all of our obsessive attention to weight-loss, cosmetics and sport, we are still in terrible condition. So what are we to do about the state of the modern human body? How can we rescue ourselves from the combined effects of stress deprivation, athletic tyranny, cosmetic obsession and physical malaise?

It is tempting to assign blame to the forces and actors that have led us to this state of physical atrophy. We could pin the blame on agriculture and fossil fuels. We could point our fingers at fashion magazine editors, weight-loss hucksters, sport marketing executives and the advertising industry. But while these forces and actors may deserve close scrutiny, such accusations may be premature.

The fundamental problem is that until quite recently, we didn't really know much about where our bodies came from. Consequently, our physical training programs have been little more than shots in the dark, wild guesses about what might improve our health and performance. Given what little we knew about our evolutionary origins, it's no wonder that our physical exercise programs were so arbitrary. Prior to the last couple of decades, we have really had very little idea of who we are or where we came from.

Before Lewis Leaky's monumental discoveries in East Africa, no one really knew much about human origins or our ancestral environment. Only the most dedicated paleoanthropologists had any idea of our roots and even these experts had only fragmentary knowledge. (And they were out digging fossils, not teaching fitness classes.) In a way, it was inevitable that we would devise ridiculously inappropriate fitness and exercise programs. We were operating almost entirely without information. Even if people wanted to practice physical training that was consistent with human evolution and physiology, there was no one out there who could tell them how to do it.

Fortunately, we have recently made some big strides in getting to know who we are and where we came from. Our modern under-standing of human ancestry began in 1859 with the publication of Charles Darwin's *Origin of Species* and his theory of natural selec-tion. Darwin's explanation was correct, but the fossil evidence for human origins was nearly nonexistent at the time and no one had any idea how physical traits might be passed from one generation to the next. Darwin guessed rightly that the origins of humanity lay in Africa, but he had little hard evidence to make his case.

Modern paleontology really began in 1925, with Raymond Dart's discovery of the "Taung child" in southern Africa. Dart claimed this find as a new genus and species—*Australopithecus africanus*. This set off a wave of interest in paleoanthropology and over the next few decades, thousands of scientists descended upon Africa, armed with shovels, toothbrushes and notebooks. Little by little, they began to fill in gaps in the fossil record. In 1974, Donald Johanson dis-covered Lucy, a nearly complete skeleton of *australopithecus* and in 1978, Mary Leaky discovered the famed fossil footprints at Laetoli, Tanzania. These incredible finds gave us a much better idea of early bipedalism and showed us that human history was both deep and complex.

While field scientists were out digging holes all across Eastern Africa, molecular biologists were hard at work back in their labo-ratories, studying the intricate structures of animal cells. DNA was first decoded in 1953 by Watson and Crick, unlocking the code of inheritance. As we studied the DNA of more and more species, we came to the astonishing realization that all living organisms use the same method to transfer genetic information from one generation to the next. We also began to understand that human beings share a great many genes with other creatures, and that in particular, we share over 98% with the chimps and bonobo. By calculating rates of mutation in the DNA molecule, we found that we could read the "molecular clock" and date major events in our evolutionary his-tory. This led to the realization that the human and great ape lines diverged roughly 6 million years ago.

Prior to the 1950's, our ideas about the age of humanity and the earth itself were wild guesses. Radiocarbon dating was first developed in 1949. Later, more advanced techniques such as the potassium-argon method enabled earth scientists to establish the age of the earth at 4.5 billion years. Increasingly accurate fossil dating techniques have given us a pretty clear picture of how old our species really is and when major events took place.

At the same time, we have come to a better understanding of our ancestral environment. Prior to the last couple of decades, we could only guess about the climate and ecology that our ancestors experienced. We could only speculate on the terrain and locomotion demands that primal peoples would have encountered. We still don't know the complete picture by any means, but we have been able to narrow it down by drilling core samples, dating sediments and looking for the presence of fossilized plants and animals. The details are still sketchy, of course, but we do have a fair idea of the terrain, climate and ecology of the primal landscape.

By bringing together hard-won facts from the fields of paleo-anthropology, molecular biology, paleoclimatology, anatomy and geology, we have at last begun to sketch out a plausible picture of what hominid life was really like, filling in the details with actual evidence and cautious speculation. Stone tools tell us about hunting and gathering practices. Fossilized teeth tell us about nutrition. Fossil bones tell us about physical stresses and diseases. Remains of non-human animals tell us about predator activity and food sources.

Taken together, these discoveries have given us a far clearer understanding of who we are. In fact, we are now living in the midst of a dramatic, unprecedented advance in human self-knowledge. Robert Ardrey, author of *African Genesis*, called this "the new enlightenment." This new understanding of human origins will change our ideas about almost everything that we say and do. It will change our ideas about politics, law, social relations, art and culture. And, of course, it will change our ideas about health, medicine and physical fitness.

There is obviously a great deal that we have yet to learn about human origins, but now, for the first time in history, we're in a position to create physical training programs that are truly congruent with who we are. Finally, for the first time in 10,000 years, we can get back into shape.

a team approach

The task before us is to start from scratch and put together a paradigm for human movement that's consistent with recent discoveries and our new understandings about who we are. For this, we're going to need an interdisciplinary approach. The body, after all, does not exist in isolation. It is not the case that we can put humans in exercise science laboratories, study them for a few years and extract precise lessons for how we ought to conduct our training programs. We are not laboratory animals, after all.

Physical health is not a single subject with a clearly-defined knowledge base. Rather, it is a broad field that spans many disciplines. When we set out to study the body, we are bound to come into contact with dozens of related and overlapping disciplines. If we really want to create an intelligent fitness program, we'll want to take an integrative, inter-disciplinary approach.

With this in mind, let's assemble a hypothetical team of experts. Let's give it an official title –The GoAnimal Council on Physical Fitness. This team will examine our physical predicament and recommend ideas, exercises and orientations for improvement. There will be three main parts of the team: the primal voices will set the context for human experience, the functionalists will study the practical elements of fitness and the playful voices will make sure we have fun in the process.

Keep in mind the fact that these voice won't necessarily agree on the specifics of particular ideas, exercises or training programs. There is simply too much diversity in this field to come to universally-endorsed conclusions. The primalists might favor a particular emphasis on field drills for example, while the functionalists might recommend a particular formula for aerobic and strength training. Nevertheless, there is consensus here and in large measure, this team is in agreement; if you adhere to these basic principles, you won't go far wrong.

Naturally, you can add other voices to the team as you wish. Depending on your own personal health and fitness objectives, you might want to include the perspectives of particular athletes, dancers, physicians or philosophers. It's up to you. As long as you keep the core orientation–primal, practical and playful–you won't go far wrong.

primal

The first part of our interdisciplinary team will be the primalists. We'll invite some biological anthropologists, paleoanthropologists, paleoclimatologists and primatologists to join us. We might also include a few contemporary hunter-gatherers, perhaps some bushmen from the Kalahari or Tanzania. These individuals will educate us about our ancestral environment and primal movement challenges. They will feed our imagination and fire our interest in what it was like to live on the semi-wooded grassland.

It is absolutely essential that we try to make our physical training consistent with human origins. We are bipedal primates, born to walk across the semi-wooded grassland, gathering, hunting and being hunted along the way. Every detail of our anatomy and physiology is adapted specifically to the demands of this kind of outdoor, multi-terrain living. If we can mimic the physical conditions faced by our ancestors, we'll give our bodies the kinds of stresses and challenges that we are adapted to. This increases the chances for fitness success.

The primalists will play a crucial role in keeping our attention on history and context. They will remind us of the vast depth of hominid history and the challenges that we have traditionally faced. They will tell us about terrain, ecology, food supplies and general living conditions. Most importantly, they will explain to us why our bodies are the way they are. And, finally, they will give us some suggestions how we can sculpt our physical training to be consistent with our heritage.

This primal orientation gives us some powerful suggestions about ways that we might create more effective and enjoyable modern lives. The fact that our bodies have been sculpted by millennia of natural selection for grassland living is compelling. Powerful as it is, we need to exercise caution with this perspective. It is very tempting to romanticize the lives of primal humans and come to conclusions that are unsupported by the facts.

It is tempting to assume that, by returning to some ancient state of nature, we'll be able to overcome our modern afflictions and find a cure for all that ails our bodies. We might even come to the conclusion that, when it comes to finding the best program for physical conditioning, "if it was good enough for *Homo erectus*, it's good enough for me."

The thing that we sometimes forget is that while primal living surely had some distinct advantages, it also included some terrible physical hardships. The grassland was a very beautiful and dangerous place. Members of your tribe would have suffered traumatic accidents, infection, illness, predator attacks and possibly even attacks by other hominid tribes. Even a completely organic diet would not change your predicament by any great measure; infant and adult mortality was probably high and life spans were short.

When we use hominid history as a means to inform and guide our modern knowledge and behavior, we inevitably run into problems of over-generalization and over-simplification. But if paleoanthropologists have learned anything over the last 50 years, it is that human history is highly diverse. Our ancestors came in many forms, lived in many different environments and practiced many kinds of behavior. Primates are highly intelligent and adaptable; they will do whatever it takes to survive. Therefore, we must be cautious when drawing conclusions based on our ancient past.

It is tempting to model our modern fitness programs on a single "hominid lifestyle," but in fact, the primal hominid lifestyle was probably included all sorts of environmental challenges and physical adaptations. Even if we could travel back in time and follow primal hominids around with a video camera, we'd probably still come up with diverse, conflicting opinions on how we ought to move. The best we can do is talk about probability. In other words, if we create a movement program that is consistent with the realities of human evolution, we'll probably get good results and have fun in the process. But we could be wrong. That's why we need to expand our understanding with other perspectives and orientations.

practical

The second part of our inter-disciplinary team includes the functionalists. These voices will keep us focused on practical considerations of modern human movement. Here we'll recruit the physical therapists, athletic trainers, kinesiologists, biomechanical specialists, podiatrists, neurologists and exercise scientists. These individuals study the precise mechanisms of human movement and the physiology of physical conditioning. They will devise exercises and conditioning programs that are consistent with modern scientific discoveries in anatomy and physiology.

The emphasis here will be on functional movement before cosmetics. For the functionalist, the way you move is more important than the way you look. High-quality movement is not only enjoyable, it also prehabilitates us against injury and gives us more options for what we can do with our bodies

This functional approach also offers the potential for dramatically improved physical performance. If you want to improve your performance in athletics, manual labor or the routine movements of daily life, functional exercises will give you the best results. By practicing specific movements that mimic the challenges you face, your body will naturally respond in the most appropriate ways. Not only that, functional exercises offer the potential for superior injury resistance and faster rehabilitation. Because they are consistent with our evolutionary heritage, functional movements tend to strengthen us in exactly the right areas that will give us the best injury resistance.

playful

The final part of our team is the playful contingent; imagine, if you will, a hypothetical pack of 8 to 12 year-old movement consultants. These voices will keep us focused on the merits of play and make sure that we don't get too serious about what we're doing. They will remind us that, regardless of what we discover about evolution, biomechanics, physiology or the merits of sets and reps, the ultimate goal is pleasure and happiness. Our young consultants will serve as a check and balance on the others, especially when they tend towards excess gravity.

By taking the child's perspective, we apply the "kid test" to the various movements and programs that we are trying to evaluate. As you have probably observed, most of today's exercise and conditioning programs are simply not very fun. On the contrary, most of them are sheer labor (that's why we call them "workouts").

Kids know what's fun and what's boring; their bodies are wired for play. That's why they will always choose a skateboard over a weight machine. They'll choose bouncy, wild movement over monotonous repetition any day. Kids hate stationary bikes; they want real bikes that they can ride around in the fresh air. They want toys with risk, things that will crash if piloted improperly.

As adults, our mistake is that we spend too much time looking for the scientifically correct, biomechanically advanced, superstar-approved training program, and not enough time going wild on the playground. If our exercise classes were actually designed to be fun, people would keep doing them.

From an evolutionary point of view, beginning an exercise program with play makes perfect sense. Young animals are genetically programmed to practice movements that are most important for their developing bodies. What's more, their bodies are rigged with positive feedback loops that reinforce movements that are appropriate for their species. When they execute these movements, they experience a pleasurable sensation known as "fun." In this respect, children's movement preferences have a legitimate place physical education.

Not only is play pleasurable, it is also highly functional. Young animals find play enjoyable precisely because those movements are appropriate for their bodies and their development. If an exercise is not fun, it is quite likely that it is not appropriate for your body either. True, there are times when we ought to push against unpleasant sensation, but play remains a vital element.

Training programs are only useful if they are actually used; therapeutic movement only works if people actually do it. An exercise program might be physiologically sound and biomechanically correct in every detail, but that means nothing if there is no pleasure in the process. The movements that we do must be intrinsically rewarding; otherwise we will find other things to do in our lives.

When we emphasize play as a foundational element in human movement, we get away from the means-to-an-end philosophy that afflicts so many weight-loss and medical-exercise programs. In this paradigm, playful exercise is pursued as an end in itself. This orientation keeps our motivation strong. Instead of looking for some future reward that may or may not come our way, we lace up our shoes for the simple fact that it feels good. When we put the emphasis on function and fun, we go a long ways towards making fitness sustainable and satisfying.

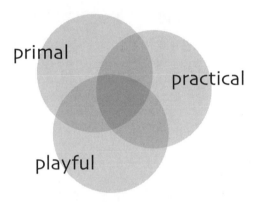

In general, the primal, practical and playful voices on our inter-disciplinary team are complementary to one another. That is, exercises that are relevant to primal conditions are likely to be practical and fun as well. Of course, the voices won't always agree with one another about the merits of any particular exercise or fitness method, but that's the beauty of it. These perspectives serve as checks and balances on one another.

The nice thing about having an interdisciplinary team on this project is that we can't go too far wrong in choosing what we do with our bodies. If the primalists get carried away with hunting, gathering and esoteric bush skills, the functionalists can bring them back into the modern world. And if the functionalists get overly obsessed with charting sets and reps on spreadsheets, the playful voices can remind them that we need to keep the fun in function.

Primal:
fitness in an
evolutionary context

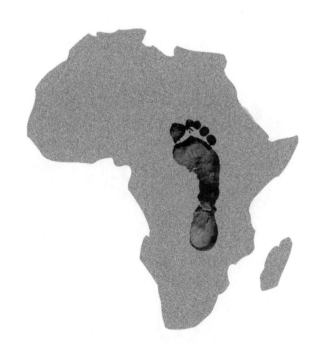

We are animals

By exploring the animal kingdom, we have found that the continuities are far more dramatic than students of evolution ever expected. The differences are of scale and degree, not of kind.

Rick Potts
Humanity's Descent

The question of whether we descended from apes, or split from apes, no longer arises, because it hasn't yet happened......We are apes.

Richard Leakey
from *The Hominid Gang*
by Delta Willis

If we're going to study fitness and exercise, we're going to have to study physiology and if we're going to study physiology we're going to have to study biology and if we study biology, we're going to have to study evolution and if we study evolution, we're going to have come to grips with the simple fact that human beings are animals. Like it or not, we are kin with every other striding, crawling, squirming, flying and swimming thing on the planet. We share many characteristics and much of our DNA coding. We are vulnerable to the same things that afflict every other creature—starvation, predation and disease to name a few. Like it or not, we are flesh and blood creatures living in a biological world.

The case for humans-as-animals is overwhelming. We now know that humans have a huge genetic overlap with all other creatures. Our physiology is unique in some details, but is substantially identical to other mammals and primates; we have a 98% genetic overlap with chimps and bonobo. We are, as Desmond Morris put it in his 1967 book of the same name, *naked apes*.

Human supremacists like to point to our big brains as proof of some kind of superiority, but a highly convoluted cerebral cortex is simply a biological adaptation, not an exemption. To say that humans aren't animals because they have big brains is like saying that vertebrates aren't animals because they have backbones. Human supremacists also like to boast that we have achieved the highest level of physical complexity and neurological sophistication but in fact, we can't even lay claim to having the most complex set of genes. The rice plant has about 100,000 genes. Humans, on the other hand have something on the order of 40,000, roughly the same number as the squid.

Denial of our animal status is becoming more difficult to maintain with each passing day; most of our precious objections have been shown to be of little consequence. Chimps use tools. They have culture. They can use sign language. They hunt. They feel pain, loneliness and pleasure. They cheat, steal, rape and murder. Even crows use tools.

In biological reality, there is no substantive difference between humans and non-human animals; we are all members of the kingdom *Animalia*. This is not to say that there are no differences between humans and non-human animals. Obviously there are differences between *Homo sapiens* and other creatures, just as there are differences between grizzly bears and pine trees. All species are unique; that's why we call them species. Yes, humans have some astonishing traits, but so do bats and killer whales. Uniqueness does not mean separation, nor does it mean superiority.

Some two thousand years ago, the Taoist philosopher Chuang Tzu wondered if "the words of men are any different than the chirping of birds." Today's biologist, equipped as he is with a broad understanding of the natural world and an appreciation for species diversity, will reply that, in one basic sense, they're not. We grope for some sort exception or exemption, but in the end, there's just no getting around the fact that we are part of the animal kingdom.

we are hominids

Not only is it correct to describe ourselves as animals, it is also correct to describe ourselves as hominids. A hominid is simply an erect-walking primate. Hominids may or may not have big brains, they may or may not use tools, they may or may not hunt game, but they all get around on two legs. There have been dozens of hominid species on the planet over the last several million years; today only one remains.

In the popular imagination, we tend to think of hominids as primitive, slouching, sub-humans of low intelligence. We think of the hominid as a "missing link" with all of the lower instincts and none of the higher refinements that characterize humans. Due to our preoccupation with *Homo sapiens*, many of us tend to think of our ancestors as inferior, less-refined versions of ourselves. We often use the term "primitive" as a pejorative, supposing that our ancestors spent their days grunting at one another and cursing their fate for not being more like us.

But from a biological point of view, this orientation turns out to be entirely incorrect. Many hominid species were highly successful and quite well-adapted to their surroundings. Some of them thrived on the grasslands of Africa for millions of years. These creatures did not lament their condition nor did they dream of one day becoming human; they had their own lives to live. It is true that our hominid ancestors had smaller brains than modern *Homo sapiens*, but in the context of evolution, this is a mere detail.

For the purpose of studying physical fitness, brain size is actually pretty irrelevant. It is our bipedal locomotion that is most relevant to human ancestry. This is why anthropologists refer to the hominids as "the human family." As Richard Leaky put it in *The Origin of Mankind*, "The origin of bipedal locomotion is so significant an adaptation that we are justified in calling all species of bipedal ape 'human.'"

From a health and fitness standpoint, we gain a great deal when we view ourselves as hominids. Instead of emphasizing differences, we emphasize the shared characteristics and common challenges that have been faced by all hominids throughout history. Yes, we have big brains, but we are still bipeds who are adapted to terrestrial life on the semi-wooded grassland of sub-Saharan Africa. If you lived deep in prehistory, you would have shared your territory with other hominid species, each with their own set of adaptations. Your big brain might have given you an advantage, but not necessarily so.

By calling ourselves hominids, we continually refresh our memory of our origins and keep ourselves in context. This orientation shapes our health and fitness behaviors and keeps them congruent with our history. It helps us to create games and exercises that are appropriate to our bodies.

life in the bush

Those who resist the suggestion that humans are animals often make their case by describing evolution as a sequential process that aims towards ever-increasing refinement and progress, ultimately expressed in the form *Homo sapiens.*

This orientation is usually illustrated as a left-to-right series of images. On the left, we have the knuckle-dragging, slack-jawed ape, a primitive creature of the distant past. Gradually, through a series of progressive "refinements" and "improvements," this creature begins to stand up, lose his body hair, walk erect and generally get his act together. Finally, in the right-hand illustration, he achieves final status as a well-groomed, culturally-sophisticated *Homo sapiens.*

This illustrated sequence appears in thousands of textbooks, newspapers and magazines all over our planet, reinforcing our belief that we are the logical end-result of millions of years of evolution. Yes, our ancestors may have been animals, but we have transcended this heritage and achieved a higher status.

The problem with this picture is that evolution simply does not work this way. What we see in the fossil record is not a linear sequence of progression towards a single, higher organism. It is not a pyramid or a ladder of progress. Rather, what we see is a flowering diversification of animals and plants, a branching bush of life. Evolution is in the business of diversification and innovation. We are one leaf on one twig on one branch.

As the late Stephen Jay Gould so often reminded us, nature produces species the way plants produce branches, shoots and leaves.

Growth of the bush takes place not in sequence, but in many directions simultaneously, wherever opportunity exists. All of the branches and leaves are dynamic and exist in a state of transition. Any branch or leaf may be pruned back by environmental forces such as food shortage, climate change or asteroid strikes.

Because words on the page come at us in a linear sequence, we sometimes get the impression that the species leading to *Homo sapiens* also came in a linear sequence. We think "First there was a common ancestor which led to *australopithecus*, which led to *Homo habilis*, which led to *Homo erectus*, which led to *Homo sapiens*."

In fact, the evolutionary process leading to humans has been messy, overlapping and above all, bushy. At any given time in prehistory, there were several different species of hominids living and interacting with one another. There was variation within tribes and between tribes.

For a long time, we thought that we could just go back, dig fossils and reconstruct the rungs on the ladder that led to *Homo sapiens*. But now we're starting to realize that this whole enterprise is far more complex than any ladder. We're mapping an immense, intertwined thicket of branches, twigs, shoots and offshoots.

what this means for health and fitness

The fact that humans are animals is not just a philosophical curiosity to be discussed in coffee shops and university lecture halls. Rather, it has profound, far-reaching implications for the way that we approach health and fitness. When we study the full scope of biology and physiology, it becomes obvious that those things that contribute to the health of non-human animals are likely to contribute to our health as well. Their bodies are substantially similar to our own. Those things that keep them vigorous and vibrant will keep us vigorous and vibrant too. Similarly, those things that adversely affect the creatures around us are likely to make us ill as well.

Human supremacists diligently police the species boundary, making lists of how we're superior to the non-human creatures around us. This is not a harmless exercise in self-promotion, however. If we insist on divorcing ourselves from the rest of the natural world, we are likely to miss important elements that contribute to our health and fitness. By creating an artificial divide, we separate ourselves from an immense body of knowledge that can provide substantial health and fitness benefits. Promoting human supremacy may make us feel good in the short run, but in the long run it will make us feel worse.

Denying our animalhood keeps us out of contact with forces, processes and experiences that keep us healthy, as individuals and as groups. And, since the natural world is the source of our life, health and fitness, denying our status as animals is like cutting off our own air supply. Yes, we can deny our membership in the animal kingdom, but we do so at our peril. If we build a pedestal for ourselves, we lose contact with a wealth of knowledge and experience that will keep up strong and healthy.

When we admit our membership in the animal kingdom, we find that we can suddenly take advantage of an immense body of knowledge that comes to us from fields such as wildlife biology, veterinary medicine, primatology and zoology. Everything that we know about non-human animals can benefit us as well. Everything we learn about primate physiology applies to us. Every discovery we make about mammalian nervous systems, immune systems and musculoskeletal systems applies to us. There is little to be lost here, and much to be gained.

Rejection of animal status is actually a perilous step towards ill-health. In fact, it would not be a stretch to interpret our current physical crisis in just this way. In other words, it's not the cars, chairs and couches that are dragging us down into an epidemic of physical atrophy; rather, it's our cultural insistence that we are separate from the rest of creation. Denying our status as animals is killing us. Similarly, it is the embrace of our animal status that will get us back on the path to health and fitness.

There is more to this than the health and fitness of out physical bodies, by the way. The way we rank ourselves in relation to the creatures around us also has implications for our psychological well-being and even our spiritual life. Attempts to deny our animalhood lead to a profound sense of spiritual isolation.

If there is something wrong with being an animal, then the whole of creation is also wrong and we are suddenly very lonely. As E.O.

Wilson has written, "We are a biological species who will find little ultimate meaning apart from the remainder of life." As it stands, we attempt to palliate this sense of loneliness by redoubling our attention to all things human, or with entertainment, drugs, or distraction. But these always fail, and we are left looking at each other wondering where our family is. As Paul Shepard put it in *The Subversive Science*, "The rejection of animality is a rejection of nature as a whole." Self-imposed isolation does us no good.

East side story

When we set out to design a fitness method that's consistent with human origins, we're obligated to learn some of the facts about how we've evolved over the last six million years. We'd like to know who are ancestors were, how they behaved and what kind of environment they lived in. Unfortunately, this can be a particularly devious and intricate task. The study of paleoanthropology is multi-disciplinary, multi-layered and just plain complicated. To understand the complete picture of human origins, we'd need to be adept in geology, ecology, anthropology, anatomy, physiology and a host of other disciplines. *National Geographic* once claimed that the study of human origins is akin to "throwing a dozen jigsaw puzzles out onto a table without having a picture to refer back to."

In spite of the tremendous difficulties, paleontologists have managed to come up with a plausible explanation for how we got here. They have combined fossil discoveries with environmental, climatological and geological data to form a picture that is plausible, although far from complete. Naturally, there is a lot of argument over the details, but nevertheless, there seems to be a broad consensus for the explanation that has come to be called the "East Side Story."

This epic story begins some 10 million years ago with rumblings deep inside the earth. At that time, most of Africa was covered by a homogeneous blanket of dense forest, home to many species of tree-dwelling primates. Things might have remained in this state of equilibrium for a long, long time, were it not for a great shifting of tectonic plates. The Somali Plate, a huge mass of crust underlying East Africa and part of the Indian Ocean, began to drift eastward, tearing the African continent in a distinct line running from North to South; this event produced the famous Rift Valley as well as a line of peaks and volcanoes.

Not surprisingly, this geologic event had substantial ecological consequences all across Eastern Africa. Specifically, changes in terrain initiated a profound transformation in regional patterns of rainfall and vegetation. The mountains created a rain shadow effect and the forest habitat began to thin out to the east of the rift. This drying and cooling climate created an ecosystem we now call "the semi-wooded grassland." In geologic terms, this transformation took place almost overnight; suddenly, a new habitat became available for exploitation by any creatures that could manage it.

As the forests dwindled, food resources became more dispersed. If you wanted to eat in this new habitat, you would have to cross open ground, traveling between groves of trees and other food-bearing plants. The tree-dwelling primates weren't well-suited to the job however. Their bodies were adapted to an arboreal existence; they could make a good living in the concentrated, food-rich forest habitat, but if forced onto open ground, they would struggle with the greater distances, heat and exposure. Their locomotion was not particularly efficient on this kind of terrain and they couldn't really cover much ground. Those who attempted such feats were rapidly eliminated from contention, either starving to death or being picked off by predators.

But among their numbers was a group, slightly different in physical structure, that was up to the task. These primates, later to be called the hominids, had a different genetic make-up that conferred upon them a slightly different bone structure than their relatives. A change in hip angles allowed the center of gravity to pass over the foot, which in turn allowed them to walk bipedally. These creatures could still climb and forage in the trees if they chose to do so, but they could also travel in the gaps between trees, gathering the various foods that grew there. This turned out to be a tremendous windfall because it allowed them to exploit an essentially empty habitat with scarce competition. There was food out there for the taking, and because they could walk further than their arboreal cousins, they could make a decent living.

The hominids flourished in the semi-wooded grassland and diversified into several species, some of which prospered for millions of years. As populations became established, other physical changes appeared. Bipedalism became firmly established. For reasons not yet fully understood, one of the hominids evolved a larger brain. This greater cognitive capacity allowed for the development of stone tools and mastery of fire. His bipedal gait allowed him to embark on a vast migration, first through the Middle East and Central Asia, then later to every corner of the planet.

The East Side Story is a convincing and highly plausible explanation, but the actual story is turning out to be more complicated than we thought. Recent discoveries have sparked a new round of re-examination; a hominid find in Central Africa is forcing us to widen our thinking. Nevertheless, we do have a reasonable outline to go on. East Side story is probably sketchy and incomplete, but it does give us enough guidance to make reasonable assumptions about the main events in human history. There can be no question that the tectonic-climactic-ecological chain of events played a big role in hominid evolution. We are children of our environment.

The home bioregion

To understand our instincts, we must turn backwards and place our minds in habitat.

Nancy Etcoff
The Science of Beauty

Like it or not, we are all Africans. Your skin may be light or dark and your hair may be straight or wavy. You may short or tall, muscular or slender. It doesn't matter. Africa is the home bioregion, the land where we took our first steps. We cannot possibly hope to understand ourselves, our physical capabilities or our health unless we study the land, terrain and ecosystem of our origins. If we can create a picture of our ancestral home, we've got a better chance of devising training programs and exercises that are appropriate for our bodies.

Ideally, we would travel to the land of our origins–the ancestral environment–and study its characteristics. Of course, East Africa today is not what it was when humans first evolved several million years ago. The land, the vegetation and the creatures have all changed, just as they have been changing throughout our evolution.

Nevertheless, there are some good clues that tell us what our ancestral environment was really like. The fossil record tells us what kind of animals lived in various regions at different times; this gives us clues about vegetation. We can look at fossilized teeth of herbivores and learn whether animals were grazing on grass or browsing on leaves. We can take core samples that tell us about pollen concentrations; these can tell us more about vegetation. We can take core samples of arctic ice which will tell us about global climactic changes. And we can even look at variations in the earth's orbit and fluctuations in the sun's energy output. Taken together, these methods give us some highly suggestive clues about the characteristics of our ancestral bioregion.

There are other clues that we can take from our own bodies. We know for example, that the human body has two mechanisms for cooling itself. Bare skin and copious sweat glands add up to highly efficient means for combating heat. We naturally assume some evolutionary purpose for this capability. That is, our ancestral environment was probably pretty warm on average, and we probably exercised a good deal.

So, while we can't say with precision exactly what our ancestral environment was like, we can at least bracket our thinking by establishing limits on probable conditions. For example, we can say that our ancestral environment did not include glaciers, heavy snowfall, tundra or long periods of darkness. At the other end of possibility, we can say that the ancestral environment probably did not include vast areas of unrelenting, super-arid desert, although there may have been extended periods of drought.

Given inevitable climate fluctuations, there were probably swings between both climactic poles. During the 6 or 7 million years of hominid evolution, conditions in Africa must have oscillated across a range—sometimes cool and damp, other times arid and scorching. Sometimes heavily forested, other times predominantly grassland. If we throw out the extremes, we are left with a reasonable guess as to what the typical ancestral environment was truly like: the semi-wooded grassland. Patches of forest and clearings, brushy hillsides and some wide open grasslands; we have little trouble picturing this environment in our minds. Often hot, sometimes cold and wet, highly diverse terrain, flora and fauna. Home—the primal playground.

the magic of mosaics

It's tempting to focus our attention on a single type of ancestral landscape, but actually, the land of our origins was probably not a homogenous ecological region. Rather, it was a mosaic of micro-habitats that coexisted side by side. During the Paleolithic, East Africa was a region of intense geologic and volcanic transformation. The earth's crust was highly active throughout this period, continually rising, sinking and breaking into fragments. Volcanoes and lava flows rearranged the landscape which in turn led to complex arrangements of water and vegetation. If we could have flown over our ancestral homeland in a light aircraft, we would have seen a jigsaw puzzle of terrain types, with grasslands, river valleys, forest and scrubby brush land alternating in an irregular patchwork arrangement. It must have been an incredibly rich landscape.

If you belonged to a tribe of early bipeds, it is highly unlikely that you would have lived in an ecological monoculture. Rather, your daily hunting and gathering experience would probably have taken you over several kinds of terrain and through diverse pockets of vegetation. Your tribe may have preferred one type of terrain or hunting area, but contact with other ecological regions would have been inevitable. The world would have been extremely rich with diverse plants and animals.

Naturally, the locomotion demands in this mosaic environment would have varied tremendously. On any given day, you would have walked–barefoot of course–through tall grass, mud or dry, rocky soil. You might have encountered thorn bushes and sandy slopes. Your tribe would have had to navigate dry river beds one season and cross swift, muddy rivers the next. Consequently, your feet, ankles, knees and hips would have been forced to make constant adjustments to compensate for these variations in terrain. Today, physical therapists recognize such diverse terrain challenges as physically therapeutic; different surface textures and shapes stimulate the sensory and motor nervous system, keeping it awake and responsive.

While some hominid tribes may have preferred particular regions, the mosaic habitat would have favored generalists who could travel widely across the landscape, over dirt, mud, sand, swamps, hills and grasslands. Such a mosaic environment would also have stimulated intelligence in the hominids. Navigating a diverse landscape places high cognitive demands on any creatures that attempt it. A well-developed cerebral cortex is a tremendous asset in cases like this; the ability to create mental maps of mixed terrain allows one to range over a wide area and still return to areas of safety and food resources. This greatly enhances one's survival potential. And, if you're good at navigating a mosaic environment, you might live long enough to make it to reproductive age, thus passing your genes into the future.

Not surprisingly, modern humans continue to find mosaic landscapes both beautiful and fascinating. As we travel from one microhabitat to another, we're struck by the changes in temperature, humidity, soils, plants and animal life. Every pocket of vegetation holds another potential surprise. Not only are mosaics inherently interesting, it seems likely that they would stimulate curiosity and intelligence. This is true not only in the short term, but it may have been an important element in human evolution as well. While monoenvironments tend to reward specialists, mosaic terrain tends to reward intelligent generalists.

It comes as no surprise that, even in the modern era, we still find mosaic landscapes and environments attractive. Our biophilic, nature-loving brains favor diverse terrain, flora and fauna. We flocked to California, not only for the warm weather, but also because the mosaic coastal range felt familiar and comfortable. We found it to be biologically and visually attractive. Similarly, we also feel comfortable in the mosaic landscape of many urban parks and university campuses. Almost without exception, these areas resemble miniature mosaic grasslands; small stands of trees with minimal underbrush, separated by broad lawns and occasional ponds. It can hardly be coincidence that they make for pleasant walking. Mosaics promise diversity and that means food and easy bipedal living; just what we want. It is easy to relax in this kind of environment.

Mosaic environments also stimulate our desire for exploration. With a rich diversity of terrain, plants, animals and hominids in every direction, we would have been intensely curious to see the sights. Even in times of abundant food and good weather, human tribes would have probably walked great distances just out of the simple desire to see the neighborhood. Mosaics stimulate wonder.

habitat generalists on the go

Not only did ancient humans thrive in the mosaic grasslands of East Africa, they also found a way to survive in a multitude of environments across the planet, all the way from Olduvai to Patagonia. As we expanded our range, we came into contact with a wide spectrum of terrain and habitat types and found a way to survive in many of them. We adapted to the hot and dry conditions of the Middle East, the cold, wet and mountainous terrain of Europe, the outback of Australia, the marine environment of the Pacific and the forests and plains of the Western Hemisphere. By making this great trek around the world, we proved that we are habitat generalists; we can function effectively across a broad range of temperatures, terrain, vegetation and variations in food supply.

Habitats inhabited by humans now include temperate grassland, forests, savanna, rain forest, deserts scrublands, mountains, swamps and mangroves, oceanic islands, polar as well as urban and suburban environments. Our ability to inhabit these diverse habitats is obviously due in large measure to our social, cultural and technological inventions; we've got tools, language and tribal cohesion to protect us. Nevertheless, our ability to live in diverse habitats is also due to the raw physical characteristics of our bodies. We can tolerate wide fluctuations in altitude and latitude. Even without our technological insulation, we can survive in regions that are hot, cold, wet or dry. In other words, we are a kind of all-terrain species.

Similarly, we know other creatures that are habitat generalists. The wolf and the grizzly bear once ranged all across North America, surviving extremes of latitude, temperature and altitude. Dogs and coyotes are incredible habitat generalists as well. In contrast, other creatures are best characterized as habitat specialists. These animals thrive within a narrow range of environmental conditions. Rainbow trout flourish in clear, cold water; but if transplanted into streams or lakes that are slightly warmer or more saline, they die almost immediately. Creatures of the deep ocean can live no where else.

From a fitness and performance point of view, this is a fundamental consideration. If you're a trainer of animals—human or non-human—you really want to take the creature's habitat preferences into account. It doesn't make any sense to train habitat generalists and specialists in the same fashion. If you're working with a specialist, you want to stay within their natural environmental range, and maybe push the comfort zone on occasion, just in case. If you're working with a habitat generalist on the other hand, you'll want the training to be more environmentally holistic; you'll want to train them for competence across the entire range of conditions that they are likely to encounter.

For humans, this means training for hot and cold, high and low, rocky and sandy, steep and level. By training people as habitat generalists, we're more likely to devise exercises and activities that are appropriate for their bodies (and their minds). And at the same time, we're less likely to create injuries. In contrast, what we are currently doing in modern fitness programs is training humans as if they were extreme habitat specialists. We put them in climate-controlled gyms and studios with perfectly level floors or on obsessively groomed athletic fields. We feed them ultra-precise combinations of refined substances at precise intervals. We have even taken to housing marathon runners in pressurized dwellings that allow them to "sleep high and train low." Then we train them to perfect an extremely narrow range of movement specialties that in many cases, don't occur anywhere else except the gym or the sporting arena. This is like taking a dog or a coyote and training it to perform on one kind of terrain, at one temperature and with a single style of movement. If you were to take such a creature and release it into the wild, it would probably die in short order.

Habitat generalists need a diversity of skills, a range of fitnesses. It's not enough to be strong or endurant in one event or one movement specialty. The grassland will challenge us in myriad ways, and the demands can change from hour to hour and even minute to minute. You might be good at one thing, but the grassland demands many things. If you want to survive for very long, you've got to be a physical generalist. As Robert Heinlein once put it, "Specialization is for insects."

Ancestral athletics

When we think about physical fitness and performance today, we generally think of popular sports and in particular, the modern Olympics, which began in 1898. As sports fans sitting in the pub, some of us are likely to ask, Who's better? Today's modern athletes or our hunting and gathering ancestors?

Many of us will reflexively suppose that our finest physical performances have come in the last one hundred years and especially in the last thirty. This perception is built on the observation that world records continue to improve in many sports, and that today's athletes are capable of far more audacious performances than those of recent past. And, if today's athletes are so much better than those of the previous generation, it goes without saying that they must also be better than our primal ancestors of the Pleistocene. Right? Surely Shaquille O'Neal could mop the floor with any *australopithecus*, *homo erectus* or *neanderthal*.

Actually, the truth would probably surprise us. Yes, records for sporting performance have improved steadily in recent decades and we can safely assume that few humans of any age would be able to match the elite, specialized performances of today's Olympians. But the thing we need to keep in mind is that this age of modern sport, audacious as it is, represents only a tiny fraction of human history. Even the 100 year history of the modern Olympics is just a miniscule percentage of human athletic experience.

Prehistory accounts for the vast, overwhelming majority of human life. It is safe to assume there must have been outstanding, epic physical performances throughout this time, that long period of hunter-gatherer life that lasted some six million years. We can also assume that our ancestors ran long distances, out-maneuvered dangerous predators and performed incredible acts of physical endurance and strength. They were wild animals, after all.

Of course, there are no surviving records of ancestral athletic performances; we have no record books for the Pleistocene epoc (1.6 million to 10,000 years ago). We don't know how fast human beings ran, how much they could lift or how gracefully they moved. Nevertheless, we can safely assume that during that long period of time, there must have been millions of cases of athletic excellence.

We can also be sure that not one of these individuals trained on chrome-plated weight machines, took vitamin supplements or counted sets and reps. Yes, they probably had shamans, herbs and superstition; they may have even engaged in strange and exotic training practices. But in general, these humans excelled on their own merits, without personal trainers, magazines, videos or programs. Clearly, physical fitness is something we are inherently capable of. It is part of who we are.

For the hunting and gathering hominid, athletic performance was not some exceptional capacity to be demonstrated on special occasions in front of assembled crowds. Rather, it was a routine, ordinary act. Every tribe member, hunter or not, had to be something of an athlete. Even the humble gatherer needed strength and endurance to travel the grassland, collect food and escape predation. Athletic competence was not some special quality bestowed on the physically gifted; it was a normal part of human experience. In short, you were either an athlete, or you were dead.

For all we know, our primal ancestors were even more athletically impressive than today's stars. The hominids had roughly the same bipedal bodies as we do today, but their training was, in a sense, technically perfect. Their lifestyle oscillated in a cycle of vigorous activity and rest. Walk a lot, rest a lot. Run then rest. Eat a little, rest. Hunt and feast, dance and rest. With this kind of low-stress, high-contrast oscillation, it is inevitable that many of the hominids would have developed prodigious physical powers. Yes, we can be sure that some hominids were forced into overtraining by bad weather, food scarcity, predators or wildfires. We can also be sure that other hominids lucked out and were able to slack off and atrophy in some friendly and fertile valley. But in the main, we can be sure that most of them developed a respectable athleticism without even trying.

What is fitness?

With all this talk about evolution, health and physical movement, it's inevitable that we will come up against the word "fitness." The average exerciser assumes that he knows what this means, but the reality is actually pretty complicated. Typically, most of us use a vague set of criteria to determine whether or not we're "in shape" or "physically fit." Being visual creatures, we tend to look first at appearances; well-toned, hard bodies are declared "fit," soft and flabby bodies are declared "unfit." Or, if we're into data, we look for a set of numbers to tell us whether or not we measure up to a particular standard.

Of course, some of us get really confused right at the outset because biologists also use the word "fitness." This causes no end of confusion. When we hear biologists talk about "survival of the fittest" we tend to assume that animals survive in the wild because of their ability to move and run like our favorite athletes. Yes, lots of non-human animals are strong, fast and agile, just like great human athletes, but this is not what biologists are talking about.

For the biologist, "fitness" refers to the overall relationship of the organism to its environment. The animal's "fit" to the environment or habitat may have nothing at all to do with its athleticism, speed, power or strength. An animal or species might be considered well-adapted or "fit" because of its ability to retain heat, digest certain plants, see in the dark, function without water or hide from predators.

When biologists talk about "survival of the fittest," they are not talking about animals with rippling muscles, awesome physiques or low body fat percentages. Instead, they are talking about a set of physical traits that allow a species to live to reproductive age and generate viable offspring. Thus, a capable immune system, a good nose or the ability to hear low-frequency sound may have as much to do with fitness as speed or strength. This means that we've got to be careful about how we phrase our objectives; if you say that you're "into fitness," it's best to be precise.

what the treadmill test tells us

In popular use, we often use the word "fitness" to describe a mix of physical qualities that include strength, endurance and flexibility as well as general health and vigor. If we're familiar with health and exercise science, we might look at some physiological criteria to tell us whether or not we're "fit." We might measure blood pressure, body-fat percentage and aerobic capacity, especially the legendary VO_2 max. We'll put you on a treadmill, straps some sensors on your chest and stick a breathing apparatus over your mouth. We'll come up with a set of numbers, compare them against other humans in your age group and, if you're on the right side of the bell curve, we'll pronounce you "fit." Good numbers mean good fitness.

As it turns out, these numbers may not mean very much. Consider this landmark study reported in the March 14, 2002 issue of the *New England Journal of Medicine.* Researchers tested and followed a group of over 6,000 men, average age 59. At the outset of the study, the researchers gathered routine medical data and tested for peak exercise capacity on the treadmill. Individuals were then followed for 6 years. During that period, some 20% of the men died. After reviewing the data, researchers found that next to age, the best predictor of mortality was peak exercise capacity on the treadmill test. The results were fascinating:

> In both healthy subjects and those with cardiovascular disease, the peak-exercise capacity achieved was a stronger predictor of an increased risk of death than clinical variables or established risk factors such as hypertension, smoking, and, diabetes as well as other exercise-test variables…

> …a man's peak exercise capacity as measured on a treadmill test is a powerful predictor of how long he will live, a predictor more powerful than estab-

lished risk factors such as hypertension, smoking, or high cholesterol.

In other words, if you've got the capacity to go long and hard on an uphill-slanting treadmill, you're probably going to live a long time, regardless of what the other numbers say. Conversely, if you've got good cholesterol, blood pressure and body fat numbers but flounder on the uphills, you may not really be in such good shape after all. It's function that matters.

As the importance of functional fitness becomes more widely recognized, we can expect it to become an integral part of medical practice. Instead of basing the annual physical exam exclusively on blood pressure and other routine measurements, physicians may find more significance in what their patients can actually do with their bodies. Eventually, the treadmill may become a pivotal diagnostic tool.

Significantly, the study also had another interesting result. The survivors had a significantly higher body mass index than the men who died. In other words, those who were heavy and fit lived longer than those who were skinny but out of shape. So, as we are beginning to see, data doesn't tell us as much as we might like.

what makes a good hunter-gatherer?

Physiological numbers and treadmill tests can be interesting, but if we really want to come up with a comprehensive definition of physical fitness, we'll also want to take a primal perspective and look at those characteristics that would make a good hunter-gatherer. After all, it was only a few moments ago that we were living on the grassland, making our living by foraging, scavenging, chasing and killing.

What physical qualities would contribute to our survival on the African plain? When we take this evolutionary approach, our first question about a person's fitness level is "How would they do in a primal hominid environment?" Would the condition of their bodies allow them to walk a diversity of terrain, searching for food, finding shelter and avoiding predation?

Notice that this orientation is entirely different from today's sporting and athletic ideal where we look for extremely high levels of proficiency in single movement types. In fact, those individuals that we commonly think of as good athletes wouldn't necessarily thrive in a primal environment. East Africa, after all, is a lot different than the artificial sporting environments that we have built for ourselves. Maybe Kobe Bryant would be an ideal member of your all-hominid dream team, but maybe not. In fact, most of today's athletes are highly specialized and excel primarily at a certain type of movement. There would be no guarantee that the ability to throw a baseball or swim a fast 1000 meters would be of any use in our ancestral environment.

Of course, the only way to know the true demands and proficiencies required in our ancestral environment would be to actually live a life of authentic hunting and gathering, something that today's coaches, physical therapists and trainers are unlikely to do. So, lacking the experience, we'll have to resort to thought experiments and a vivid imagination.

Set your time machine for 100,000 BC, push the button and see what it takes to survive to reproductive age and beyond. Will you need strength? How much? Flexibility? Cardiovascular fitness? Sensory acuity? Suppose you were enlisted to coach for a tribe of hunter-gatherers. How would you train them? Would you make them lift rocks? Take laps around the grassland? Dig holes? Throw projectiles? Wrestle? The way you answer these questions will suggest a possible standard for human fitness.

a hunted gatherer

When we think about the lives of primal humans, most of us fall back on the standard-issue image of man as a bold, intrepid hunter. We think of him living in caves or on the grassland, venturing forth on the hunt and returning to camp late in the day, dragging a fresh kill for the evening barbecue. We might even go so far as to explain the development of our various traits and abilities in this context— hunting challenged us to develop sociality, increased intelligence and language, for example.

But for better or for worse, we now know that this view is almost certainly an over-hyped version of human glory, a story that, for the most part, exists mostly in modern minds. Yes, we can be sure that there was some hunting going on in our ancestral past, but the practice was far more humble than we usually imagine. Our ancestors actually spent a great deal of time digging roots, scavenging from carnivore kills and trying to avoid hungry predators. We weren't the only hunters on the African plain after all.

Ken Grimes, a science writer in London, made this case in the April 13, 2002 issue of *New Scientist*. Early humans weren't chest-thumping spear-throwers as we are so quick to suppose; rather, we were one of the daily specials on the grassland menu. In describing hominid life in our ancestral environment, Grimes wrote

> What many accounts fail to emphasize is the hellish nature of this new environment. In the forest lurked saber-tooths, leopards, and giant carnivorous bears. More dangerous still was the ever-expanding savannah, patrolled by pack-hunting predators—giant flesh shearing hyenas, blade-toothed dogs the size of wolves, lions and yet more saber-tooths.

Human vulnerability to predation is something that becomes abundantly clear to any tourist who travels to modern-day Africa. The grassland is no zoo; there are no fences and the carnivores are free to go wherever they please and eat whatever they want. For the tourist who's standing next to the Land Rover, line of sight is often limited by brush and terrain, so there's really no way to tell which creatures are out there and what they're doing. Leave the Rover, walk a few yards into the bush to take a photograph and you suddenly get the true picture; you're vulnerable.

This true extent of the "prey phase" of human experience has recently been revealed to us in the fossil record. Explorations of carnivore lairs in South African caves have turned up the fossil bones of numerous baboons and *australopithecus*, many of them bearing the marks of tooth and claw by big cats and hyenas. And if *australopithecus* was on the menu, we can be sure that early *Homo sapiens* was there as well. Even today we may find the same predicament; if you're audacious enough to backpack in modern day Alaska, you'll realize that *Homo sapiens* is still very much on the menu. ("Served fresh, with a blueberry garnish.")

Modern research into patterns of carnivore predation confirms this pattern. Researchers regularly find primate remains in the droppings of large carnivores. And why not? Humans and chimps eat other primates, why shouldn't large felines also eat primates? Meat is where you find it. If you're a carnivore or an omnivore, you kill what you can.

In sum, we can boil human history down to three phases. During the long, early phase of hominid life, we were small-bodied, vegetarian hunted-gatherers. Much later, we got enough traction with sociality, big brains, tools and weapons so that we could do some genuine hunting of our own. Then, much more recently, we managed to exterminate and isolate the predators to such a degree that, with the exception of occasional field trips to Alaska and Africa, we can walk about in a state of predator-free bliss.

The fact that humans have been "on the menu" for a large percentage of our history has some intriguing implications for modern physical fitness training. When we're out for a training run, for example, it just doesn't make sense to imagine ourselves as intrepid, long-distance hunters, chasing stupid and hapless herbivores for mile after mile across the grassland. A more accurate visualization would be to imagine ourselves walking furtively through a scrubby grassland in a highly focused state of alertness, always ready to sprint, climb or if necessary, fight back. Short-term speed, wits and mobilization are fundamental here. Endurance is good too, but it may actually be of secondary importance; after all, if you don't evade the lightning-quick sprint of the leopard, it doesn't matter what other skills you have.

Today's long distance runners like to interpret human history so as to justify their sport. They claim that ultra-long distance endurance was a pivotal factor in our ability to hunt and survive. But as our knowledge of human evolution grows more complete, we can see that a diversity of locomotion skills was far more important to survival. Yes, endurance is useful when you're following herds of ungulates, but herd animals don't run marathon distances; they migrate in a stop-and-go fashion. And even if you are running after game, you can also be sure that someone is running after you. You don't avoid predation by running 10 or 20 miles. You avoid predation by knowing the land around you, keeping your eyes open, staying with the tribe and, when things get really hot, running like hell for the nearest refuge.

In *Racing the Antelope*, author Bernd Heinrich claimed that long-distance running was essential to early human survival and suggested that evolution favored those who could chase ungulate prey for mile after mile across the grassland. He points to our well-established ability to withstand high temperatures, dumping excess heat through an efficient sweating mechanism. He also cites prodigious feats of endurance running by indigenous peoples around the world.

Nevertheless, it is far from certain that ancient hominids actually hunted by running long distances; in fact, the reality is probably far more complex. For example, the famed paleontologist Louis Leaky grew up with indigenous peoples in Kenya and learned an entirely different style of hunting. On safari in East Africa, he once demonstrated this method for a visiting reporter. By cloaking himself with leaves and branches, Leaky approached a gazelle that was some two hundred and fifty yards away. After two hours of stealthy, subtle movements, Louis closed the gap to six feet and executed "a perfectly timed flying tackle." Patience and cunning yes, long-distance running endurance, no.

This story suggests that stealth and endurance are equally plausible hunting strategies. We can imagine that some tribes depended on one or the other or that they changed their methods to suit their prey, the season, the wind or the terrain. Certainly, there was no single, universal method. Rather, a diversity of abilities was the key.

When modern people think about subsistence in ancestral conditions, we are likely to imagine ourselves gathering roots or hunting animals. What we tend to overlook is the opportunistic theft and scavenging that must have taken place routinely. How much scavenging we actually did is of course difficult to measure, but it may have been significant. Scavenging is actually a highly efficient means of securing nourishment. In her book, *Ancestral Passions,* author Virginia Morell relates this story about the Leakys:

> In an effort to demonstrate that early humans may have obtained their meat by stealing as well as by hunting, Louis and his son Richard sometimes chased carnivores away from their kills. "We chased off packs of hyenas, and once we disturbed some lions on a kill, without a vehicle, just carrying our firearms to see if they'd leave," Richard recalled, "which they did."

In late 2000, I was able to spend time with the Hadza people of northern Tanzania in East Africa, known locally as "the bushmen." These people live in the arid grassland of the great Rift Valley. Anthropologists consider them to be prime research subjects for how early humans might have made their living in similar ancestral habitats. What researchers have found is that Hadza hunters adopt different hunting strategies depending on the season. In the wet season, the men go off on foraging excursions, stalking a wide range of animals and shooting them with poisoned arrows. During these hunts, the hunters are highly active, walking at a brisk pace, occasionally breaking into a run, sometimes stopping for a smoke and a chat.

In the dry season, the hunters change tactics. They wait in blinds near water holes and capture the prey that comes to drink. They also scavenge. By watching the signal flights of vultures, they locate areas where lions and other carnivores are active. Upon finding a carcass, they drive off the original owner by any means possible.

This pattern suggests that, for the Hadza at least, athletic fitness may be a seasonal affair; one kind of fitness in the dry season, another in the rainy season. Given that prey animals often change their behaviors with the seasons, we can safely assume that seasonal fitness adaptations were common in many human tribes throughout pre-history.

For modern exercisers, this idea sounds instinctively appealing. Instead of grinding out a monotonous workout schedule year-round, why not mix it up with the seasons? Maybe you'd choose to work sprints in the summer and distance in the winter, or power in the spring and agility in the fall. The prospect of physical oscillation sounds a lot more interesting and sustainable than being a mono-athlete. Not only that, if you like to train hard, you'll give yourself a rest in alternating seasons.

In any case, hunting, gathering and predator avoidance are highly complex, sophisticated behaviors that demand much more than strength or endurance. If simple strength or endurance was adequate to succeed in a primal environment, we would expect young hunters to be the most successful. In fact, this is not what we see. A study reported in the *Journal of Human Evolution* (vol 42, p639) found that, when it comes to hunting, brains may be more important than brawn. Researchers studied forest hunters in Paraguay and found that, although the physical strength of hunters peaks at about age 24, they don't really excel at bringing home the meat until they approach age 40. The older hunters bring in roughly twice the amount of meat as their younger associates. This may be a simple case of "old age and treachery overcoming youth and fitness," but it also reveals the folly of using a single sport or movement specialty as a fitness standard. The ability to excel at in one physical dimension simply doesn't mean very much.

speed trap

When we practice competitive sports, we usually look for some way to measure performance and in turn, rank individuals in a hierarchy. In running events, this simplest way to do this is by measuring speed with a stopwatch. This gives us a consistent standard for evaluation and allows us to rank individuals, but the question remains, "is speed really important?"

In terms of ancestral challenges, speed is only one consideration for success. When you're in the bush, it's simply not enough to be fast. You've got to know when to go fast, when to go slow and when to hide. In fact, going fast at the wrong time may be a complete waste of time. Even worse, it might be fatal. The good hunter may be swift, but more importantly, he chooses his moments and his pace carefully. It's easy to imagine situations in which slowing down would improve results: following a faint animal track, traveling during the heat of the day or maneuvering to avoid predators for example.

This is why today's great athletes might not do very well in primal conditions. A 2:15 marathoner can cover an astonishing amount of ground in a short time, for example, but has no experience in changing his cadence to suit environmental conditions. Because his training does not include such skills as navigation and environmental scanning, he may actually be less likely to survive the bush than less-fit but more astute colleagues.

Casual observers of the natural world often envy the speed of certain non-human animals; antelopes, horses and cheetah for example. The thing that we forget is that while speed is certainly spectacular, discretion is equally vital. High-speed sprinting is extremely taxing for any creature. It is a significant energy expenditure and exposes one to injury—not something to be undertaken frivolously. Success comes, not by simply running fast, but by running fast at the right time.

If all you think about is speed or power or some other movement specialty, you're likely to miss vital information about your environment. Like navigation, environmental scanning was a vital hominid skill throughout prehistory. The bush is three dimensional: hazards and opportunities can be to your left or right, forward or behind, high or low. For hominids, daily life was a case of "leopards above, snakes below." Such a predicament demanded a fluid, mobile scan. If you drop your scan to concentrate on any single movement pattern, you're likely to suffer a blind spot.

it's about your life

If we take a really broad, quality-of-life perspective and include things like happiness and satisfaction, we come up with some different ideas about what it means to be physically fit. What is interesting in this context are real-life abilities. In this sense, we say that a person is "fit" when he or she has the ability to do what he or she wants in life. If you have the strength, speed and endurance to do the things that you want to do, then you're fit. If you can't do what you want because of physical limitations, you're not. End of story.

Obviously, we are going to see a wide range of individual variation, subjectivity and interpretation here. If your only aspiration in life is to play billiards with your friends at the pub, your aerobic capacity, VO$_2$ max and body-fat levels are all basically irrelevant. On the other hand, if your aspiration is to climb an 8,000 meter Himalayan peak without supplemental oxygen, almost any physiological capability will be insufficient. The overall demands are so extreme that just about any level of cardio-pulmonary capability and muscular endurance will be inadequate. Sorry, but even if you train fanatically, you'll still be "out of shape."

So, instead of getting out your body fat calipers or compulsively clocking your time for a 10K, a better beginning is to give some thought to what you actually want to do with your body during your lifetime. If you haven't thought about this, then you are in no position to say whether you're in shape or not. Depending on what your goals are, you might already be in terrific shape or you might have a lot of work ahead of you. This means you've got some homework to do. Write down your physical objectives in detail. Describe the kinds of activities you want to be doing next year or in 10 years, then start your training. After a few months, reassess the state of your body in comparison to what you really want to do.

What's primal, what's not

Ideally, the exercises that we choose should have some relevance to the challenges of bipedal locomotion and our evolutionary lifestyle as hunters and gatherers. In general, this means selecting movements that enhance our ability to walk and run moderate distances over varied terrain, hunting and gathering along the way. If you can't imagine *australopithecus, Homo erectus* or ancient *Homo sapiens* benefiting from the exercise, it's probably not all that appropriate for your body.

If you can't decide whether or not an exercise is primal, take an imaginary trip in the time machine, back about 100,000 years. Will the exercise in question enhance your survival? Will it help you escape predators, find food and travel over rough terrain? Let's look at an assortment of games, sports and exercises and evaluate them for their relevance to human origins and evolutionary history.

walking

Obviously, walking is the most primal of all human movements (except sex, of course). The unfortunate thing in today's world is that we have to look long and hard to find anyone who's actually walking primally. Errand walking—the kind we do between the car and the store—hardly qualifies. Our hands are usually full and our minds are focused on the errand, not on the quality of our movement.

Treadmills don't qualify either; the biomechanics of walking on a moving belt are entirely different than accelerating your body over mixed terrain. Hiking sounds like a good candidate for primal status, but when we add heavy boots and a backpack, our biomechanics change considerably. Boots give us an entirely novel gait pattern and heavy packs turn us into well, pack animals. To walk in a way that is authentically primal, we need to have our minds free, our feet light and our bodies outdoors.

running

Running is also highly primal. Sprinting, medium-distance and long-distance abilities are all potentially useful to the hunter-gatherer. The problem comes when we take running out of it's natural context and turn it into a sport. As soon as we abstract it and start specializing, we lose some of the related primal qualities that naturally go along with grassland running—navigation, tracking, predator avoidance, prey observation—and concentrate on one single consideration: speed over a fixed distance. Ancient humans must have run all kinds of distances and speed was only one possible ingredient for success. Agility, route-finding, weather observation, tribal cohesion and stealth were just as important as time over distance. So, while we can say that running is primal, sport running ranks as less so. The more specialized the running event, the less relevance it has for human history and for modern-day fitness.

climbing

Walking and running are fundamental to who we are, but it is equally true that our origins are in the trees. Most of our primate cousins are good climbers and it's easy to imagine our hominid ancestors climbing trees and rocks to get food, escape predators or simply to get a better view of the neighborhood. The ability to climb a tree or a boulder could potentially make a big difference in survivability. Thus, it makes sense to include some kind of basic climbing movements in a basic exercise program.

Of course, today's extreme sport climbing is something else altogether. As steepness and difficulty levels increase, the sport becomes abstracted from it's primal origins and ultimately becomes an movement specialty. While our ancestors undoubtedly climbed basic terrain features such as trees and rocks, we can be sure that they avoided the extremely overhanging problems and radical movements that characterize today's sport.

dance

Dance was the first human movement not directly associated with survival challenges and reproduction and is, of course, highly primal. No record exists the earliest dance forms, but we can safely assume that early dances were either spontaneous physical expressions or mimicry of animal movements. Early dances took place outdoors and coincided with the regular cycles of tribal living. This makes dance an ideal form of exercise.

Nevertheless, we can and do get carried away. We abstract particular dance movements and create distinct, highly specialized styles. Instead of dancing on special occasions, today's dancers practice relentlessly. The modern dance world is highly competitive, no less so than professional sports. Success demands that dancers push themselves to extremes of endurance and difficulty, which in turn leads to nearly inevitable injury (dancers have an injury rate similar to professional athletes). This demonstrates the fact that even the most appropriate and natural movement types, if pushed hard enough, become dysfunctional.

gymnastics

Gymnastics seems to be a promising candidate for primal status because it demands many skills that might be useful on the grassland, especially balance, agility and core body strength. Unfortunately, these components have been extracted and distilled into a hyper-competitive sport that has little or no relevance to human origins. There were no high bars, rings or uneven parallel bars in ancient Africa. The balance beam seems like a good approximation of a log across a stream, but beyond that, gymnastics has become too specialized to be considered truly primal.

the big three

We can look at the big three sports—football, baseball and basketball—together because they are all hybrids. Some of the individual movement skills are highly primal and could easily be translated into grassland success. The powerful agility of the running back, the quick lateral movement of the shortstop and the awesome dexterity of the point guard would all be highly desirable in any tribe of hominids. But there are plenty of irrelevant movements here too: the blocking power of the lineman, the ability throw a knuckle ball and the skill to hit a three-point shot, for example. These movements can be entertaining, but it's hard to imagine that they'd have any application to grassland living.

hockey

Hockey is easy to evaluate. In all probability, there were no frozen lakes on the plains of ancestral Africa and even if there were, it's impossible to imagine that the ability to skate and shoot a puck would have contributed anything to hominid survival. If it's cold enough to freeze entire lakes, you're probably going to be huddled around a fire, not playing games. (On the other hand, the ability to beat opponents with a hockey stick could translate into hunting success.)

soccer

The ability to kick or dribble a ball has no direct relevance to grassland living, but the skills that go with it certainly do. Powerful running with quick direction changes is ideal for grassland competence. If our goal was to assemble an all-hominid dream team, we would do well to include some professional soccer players.

triathalons

Triathalons cannot be considered primal for a couple of reasons. First, there were no bikes in Paleolithic Africa. Second, swimming, if it was practiced at all, was probably a desperate matter of short-distance survival. Our ancestral environment probably included shallow lakes, murky ponds and seasonal rivers; distinctly dangerous places, filled with carnivorous reptiles. The key to survival was not the ability to swim fast over a long distance. More likely, the key was avoiding the water whenever possible, usually by finding a way around it. It's not uncommon for mammals to cross open water in search of food, and our ancestors may have done the same, but such a swim would probably be a short, heads-up effort.

dodge ball

Dodge ball advocates say that it builds character and prepares young students for the competitive rigors of the real world. Opponents claim that it is frightening and intimidating for weaker players and that it fosters aggressive behavior. Incredibly, both sides miss the central point. The question we ought to be asking is, "Does dodge ball have any relationship to the primal challenges faced by ancestral humans?"

The answer is clearly no. Only in *The Far Side* would we ever see carnivores throwing rocks at hominids and even then, the hominids would still have the option to run, hide or return fire. It is difficult to imagine a grassland analogue to dodge ball. We might suppose that tribes of hominids threw rocks and mud at one another, but it's hard to imagine that this was a significant part of the grassland experience.

If practiced regularly, dodge ball could develop left-right, frontal plane agility. This is actually an important physical skill that is part of a well-rounded program, but there are better ways to develop it. Basketball drills, stepping drills and cone courses all do the same thing, without the nonsensical use of projectiles.

hop scotch

Modern athletes consider this a game for sissies, but with a little imagination, hop scotch can be highly primal and extremely challenging. The ability to execute precise, powerful variations on bipedal locomotion are clearly relevant to hominid survival. Of course, physical educators don't need to use the straight-ahead linear box patterns that we see on so many playgrounds. We can create any kind of course we want, mapping it out with tape or paint. And it doesn't have to be flat either. It's a simple matter to integrate ups and downs into the pattern. And, it's easy to spread the course across whatever field we've got available. With a little trickery, we can incorporate skips, hops, short runs and cross-steps in thousands of combinations. In fact, if we space the steps far apart and add some elevation changes, we can easily create a killer hopscotch course that would challenge the most hard-core athletes. Physical therapists commonly use hop-scotch-like movements in their clinics to rehabilitate certain weaknesses of the ankles, knees and hips. Clearly, there is value here.

obstacle courses

Obstacle courses are obviously primal. A basic course with natural obstacles such as hills, vegetation, rocks and downed trees is supremely relevant to human origins. Unfortunately, we moderns tend to get carried away. By adding exotic challenges such as cable crossings and rope problems, we turn obstacle courses into a specialty events. And, by putting our emphasis exclusively on speed, we take away from the other terrestrial skills that are part of the total hominid package: navigation and environmental scanning. Nevertheless, obstacle courses can and should be a fundamental part of basic physical education.

jump rope

At first glance, jump rope doesn't have seem to have much direct primal relevance. The ability to float like a butterfly inside a spinning rope might win you some points with your tribe members, but the local predators and prey aren't going to be impressed. Nevertheless, the physical conditioning that comes with regular jump rope training is highly transferable to primal challenges: agility, whole body coordination and short-term power endurance would serve us well on the grassland. A good jump roper would likely be a good hunter as well. And, of course, jumping rope is really fun, especially when you've mastered the basic skills.

tag

In the game of tag, one person is designated as "it" and then tries to pass his status off onto someone else. Given the enthusiastic way that children take to this game, we can reasonably assume that there's some primal relevance here. As challenge of agility and avoidance, it builds skills that would clearly come in handy on the grassland. The "it," of course, is a predator; the goal is to escape his claws and teeth. Play this game intensively for a few years and you'd be well equipped to escape the lunge of a snake, a hyena or a hostile hominid from another tribe. Now add in some running games that are commonly played by young people and you've got a grassland-ready human body. Tag is a great game, the only problem is that we quit playing it too soon.

bench press

Bench press simply doesn't have much relevance to the ancestral human experience. No self-respecting hominid would lie on his back to lift rocks or firewood. In fact, when you live on a landscape of dirt, rocks, sticks and thorny plants, you're not going to lie down at all unless conditions are just right. Even if our ancestors did have benches and barbells in ancient Africa, it's hard to imagine that such a training program would have given them much of an advantage; proficiency in this kind of pressing movement doesn't translate very well into any hunting or gathering skill. We can say that success in the bench press wouldn't have done much for hominid survival.

bike

Quite obviously, bike riding has no relevance to our ancestral past. We have yet to see any evidence of bicycles in the fossil record and we can safely assume that bike riding had no influence on human survival or physiology. This is not to say that we shouldn't ride bikes; after all, this is one activity that is universally child-approved and is just plain fun. Plus, most bike-riding takes place outdoors, which has its own value. This is particularly the case with remote mountain-biking. In contrast, stationary, indoor bike-riding is neither primal or fun.

Frisbee

At first glance, Frisbee hardly seems like a primal game. There were no flying disks on the ancestral plains and even boomerangs didn't appear until relatively recently. Nevertheless, we can see primal value here. The basic physical elements involved in Frisbee would translate easily into grassland success. Intensive locomotion with lots of starts, stops and changes of direction, swift movements with acceleration and deceleration and peripheral awareness of your tribe members create a pretty well-rounded hominid package. Plus, it's really fun.

golf

Golf is a particularly interesting case. On the one hand, it's just another abstracted movement specialty that has little or nothing to do with any other activity actually performed by humans. The movement itself has no practical function, either historically or in modern terms. Nevertheless, golf does have a primal appeal in the way that it puts us outdoors and, unless one uses a cart, encourages us to walk. Golf can put us in more intimate contact with fresh air, plants, the sky and open water. In this sense, it is a biophilic experience. It is no accident that golf courses have an strong resemblance to mosaic grasslands, our ancestral home. It is no surprise that golf is so immensely popular.

Of course, the modern golf course only mimics the most comforting, soothing and nurturing qualities of our ancestral environment; it's a sort of grassland-lite. The trees, shrubs and ponds are there, but the predators are absent. What golf needs, more than anything, are some hungry carnivores. If golf is to be a truly authentic primal experience, we need some resident predators to challenge our locomotion and our wits. Perhaps a few mountain lions on the back nine. Think of the action. Tiger meets lion at the U.S. Open! Agusta admits women and grizzly bears!

President's Council tests

When we evaluate movements and exercises in an evolutionary context, it is essential that we also take a look at the tests administered to school children by the President's Council on Physical Fitness. Given the widespread use of these tests, we might wonder if they have any relevance to human origins.

On the primal side, the tests include a mile run/walk and a shuttle run, a test that requires students to sprint back and forth across a 30 foot course. Both of these events are highly relevant to human origins; it's easy to imagine these physical skills being put to good use in pursuit of small animals or in evasion of large ones.

But what about pull-ups? Here might imagine an extreme case in which the fate of a hominid depended on his or her ability to pull up on a tree branch. But this seems a bit of a stretch; we have to ask why the fleeing hominid isn't allowed to use his feet for climbing.

And what of the notorious curl-up? In this test, an assistant holds the student's feet to the floor while the subject crosses his or her arms across the chest and does as many reps as possible. Obviously, there's no relevance to human evolution here; hominid abdominals stabilized the body core in hunting and gathering movements, not lying in the dirt.

Finally we have the V-sit. Here the subject sits on the floor with legs straight and reaches out towards his or her toes. This movement is supposed to test flexibility of the hamstrings and lower back, but not only is it notoriously inaccurate, it has no relevance to any ancestral movement.

So, we can see that the President's Council tests are a mixed bag. There are a couple of good practical movements in the set, but in general, the process seems geared, not to students, but to administrators who are trying to collect numbers. If we really wanted to teach physical education, we'd spend more time playing primal games and less time scribbling on clipboards.

the merits of middle distance

We can also evaluate popular training methods in terms of their primal relevance. As you probably know, physical training usually involves some number of repetitions against some level of resistance. We can combine these two variables in countless ways to get different training effects, but most of us tend to group these possibilities into two basic types.

At one end of the spectrum are activities that involve low levels of resistance with extremely high numbers of repetitions. These are often described as "aerobic" or "endurance" training. The classic examples of this type are running, bicycling and long-distance swimming. The most extreme examples include the notorious Race Across America (a go-like-hell bicycle race from West to East Coast), the Tour de France and the various ultra-marathons. In these events, the resistance in each rep is low, but the repetitions number in the millions to trillions.

The advantage to this kind of training is that it burns immense numbers of calories and increases cardiovascular fitness, something that many of us can benefit from. The disadvantage is that it is incredibly boring and offers limited and diminishing functional returns. It builds extremely deep neurological ruts and movement patterns that can be difficult to break out of. If you do several billion repetitions of anything, that pattern will become etched deeply into your nervous system.

At the other end of the spectrum we find the strength and power training that involves high loads with very few repetitions. The most extreme examples are in power and Olympic lifting where contestants attempt to lift the maximum possible poundage in a single rep. For example, the Holy Grail in squatting is to do one rep with 1,000 pounds. Maximum bench press is another popular one-rep strength event.

Naturally, there is a middle ground between these two types of training, a style called power-endurance. This involves mid-range loads with a middle range of repetition, performed, not to "failure" as in conventional strength training, but to heavy fatigue. In track and field, this is the "middle distance" event such as the 880 meter run; it's not a sprint, but it's not a "run" either. Many calisthenic programs such as those used in the military emphasize power-endurance—run uphill with a pack, do as many push ups as you can, then jumping jacks until your arms fall off—these are all medium reps, medium resistance.

The merits of this kind of training are difficult to assess because they seem to go in both directions. That is, power-endurance training builds some strength and some endurance. If you do lots of reps with moderate resistance, you're going to get somewhat stronger and somewhat more endurant. Your gains will not be spectacular, but they will be solid.

Here we speculate as to which form of training is most in keeping with our hunting and gathering heritage. Would hunters and gatherers ever need extreme long range endurance to succeed on the open grassland? Probably not. It is hard to imagine a hunter-gathering tribe running for 26 miles or 100 miles. You might follow a herd of animals in a semi-sustained, stop-and-go manner for days or even weeks, but to my knowledge, no predator chases prey for anything remotely approaching 26 miles. (The 26 mile distance for the marathon is an arbitrary figure taken from Greek mythology. It has nothing whatsoever to do with any physiological objective, nor does it correlate with any activity that humans actually perform.)

Similarly, it is hard to imagine that a hunter-gatherer would ever need the equivalent strength to bench press 400 lbs or squat 600. What purpose could such power possibly serve? Sure, you might need to lift a big rock or a tree limb to build a shelter, or you might, if you're lucky, have to move the carcass of a large animal. But in general, the loads would be middle range at most: gathering rocks, digging holes and hauling firewood, for example.

In fact, if I was a tribal trainer in the Paleolithic, I'd make my athletes work really hard on the middle-distance, middle-resistance work. I make 'em run uphill to the big tree and back, rest for a minute, then do it again. Hard and fast, but not too far. The fitness adaptations they gained might not be perfectly appropriate for a demands they'd encounter next month or next year, but it would be a simple matter to change their training towards strength or towards endurance as conditions dictated.

When it comes to general prehabilitation and injury-resistance, middle distance also makes sense. If we specialize at one end of the spectrum, we'll naturally miss out on some of the benefits at the other end. Concentrate on endurance events and you'll miss the benefits that come with strength training. Concentrate on strength events and your cardiovascular system will miss out. Of course, if you're a physical omnivore and you've got lots of time, you can do both, but for most people the more practical solution is simply to train in the middle.

Here it makes sense to train broadly. Do some endurance work, some strength work and some power-endurance. If your exercise history is concentrated in one area, work in the other direction to balance out your physiology and musculoskeletal condition. Of course, if your goal is to make specific gains for a particular activity or sport, you must train with the appropriate combination of resistance and reps for that sport or activity. In any event, remember that middle resistance/middle reps does not mean that you should reduce your intensity level. Push yourself! There's a carnivore back there, and he's gaining on you.

Practical:
focus on function

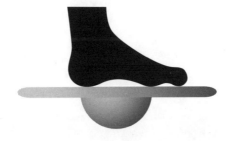

The virtues of the functional approach

These days, the hottest buzzword in physical training, athletics and rehabilitation is the word "functional." Attend a seminar of coaches, trainers or physical therapists and you're bound to hear some passionate discussions about whether or not an exercise or training practice is truly functional. Let's look into the origins of this concept and find out why it's gaining popularity.

For a long time, medicine and athletic training were entirely separate disciplines operating at opposite ends of the university campus. Medicine was basically an independent, stand-alone profession. Physicians studied the mechanisms of pathology and tried to get sick and injured people back on their feet by whatever means possible. At the other end of campus, athletic coaches were coming at the human body from an entirely different direction. They started with healthy bodies and tried to extract the highest possible physical performance from them.

For the most part, doctors and coaches didn't really talk to one another much. The conversation, such as it was, centered around rehabilitating injured athletes. Things have come a long way in the last couple of decades however, and the conversation has become more substantive. As our understanding of the human body has grown, doctors and coaches have discovered that they really have quite a bit in common.

As we might expect, coaches are now spending more time looking into sports injuries and trying to integrate modern rehabilitation and prehabilitation practices into their workouts. If your athlete is a campus star or is being paid a few million dollars a year, you'll do your research. At the same time, physicians are starting to realize that exercise is extremely powerful medicine and that coaches know a whole lot about how to apply it. If a coach can turn a set of weak legs into strong ones, he should also be able to help the physician get an injured patient back on his feet.

For years, the gap between doctor and coach has been filled by the physical therapist. During the course of his training, the PT visits both ends of campus; today's physical therapist has one foot planted in the camp of injury rehabilitation, the other in the camp of athletic performance. He is interested in physical problems such as sprains, tendinitis and post-surgical rehabilitation, but he's also interested in methods of improving strength, flexibility and endurance.

Today, these three professions are becoming increasingly united in their interest in physical functionality. Consensus is building for the view that the best exercise programs are based on practical movement skills, not on cosmetics. The promise of the functional orientation is immense. If we train people in practical, real-world movement skills, they won't be so likely to wind up in the physician's office, and if they do, they're likely to recover a whole lot faster.

isolation v. integration

Modern interest in functional training is partly a response to the exercise methodology promoted by bodybuilders over the last several decades. If you've done some strength training, you've probably heard the conventional advice that it's essential to set up your exercises to "isolate" your muscles and push them to "failure." This kind of advice has become so ubiquitous in today's gym that few people would even imagine that there's any other way to do resistance training.

Actually, there are two ways to classify human movements and exercises; we can say that they are either isolating or integrating. The difference lies in the number of muscles that are doing the work. Isolating exercises are designed to put the load on one muscle or one segment of a kinetic chain. In contrast, integrative exercises spread the load out over long kinetic chains and several muscle groups; many links in the chain participate in the movement.

Dumbbell curls, quad extensions on the machine and pectoral flys are good examples of isolation. These exercises demand maximum effort from a single muscle (or muscle group) and tend to produce strength gains in that particular area. These exercises strengthen one link in the chain. By selectively overloading one muscle, we apply the greatest possible training stimulus, inflict the greatest amount of microscopic injury and thus produce the greatest possible level of local supercompensation. In other words, we can make that particular muscle stronger.

Isolation exercises can give good, even spectacular cosmetic results, but they really don't do much for the quality of our movement. The problem is that they train us for movements that simply don't occur in the real world. If we were to do a survey of common movements performed in typical human activity–hunting and gathering, blue-collar construction, domestic labor, athletics–we would be hard pressed to find any that demand activation of a single muscle at a time. Whether you're picking up the laundry, carrying groceries or playing catch, you're usually using many muscles in coordination with one another. In the real world, we almost never perform an isolated, single-muscle movement.

If we train with a steady diet of isolationist, bodybuilding exercises, we're training ourselves to perform movements that don't occur in the real world. In other words, our training is not functional. Such training might give us some localized strength or cosmetic gains, but it won't prepare us for practical movements that we are actually going to perform.

For the modern coach, physician and physical therapist, this isolationist approach to muscular conditioning seems like a waste of time. One of the primary rules of physical training is to make practice specific to the intended outcome. But isolation isn't really specific to any real-world activity performed by humans; in other words, it's not functional.

Isolating exercises can actually be extremely counter-productive. Since they teach us to use only one muscle or kinetic link at a time, they facilitate movement patterns that are highly inefficient. A steady diet of isolation will lead to injury and poor functional performance.

It is true that today's athletes now do serious isolation work, but they usually do it in the off-season as a supplement to their regular training, never as a steady diet. Integrative, whole-body exercise remains the staple for athletic training; it is safe to say that no one has ever achieved athletic success on a program of pure isolation. It is also the case that serious bodybuilders never succeed in athletics, unless they completely revamp their training.

For the functionalist, complete integration of the body is the ultimate goal. Teach your whole body to participate in the movements you make; distribute the load across your entire body. Instead of using just your arms to lift something, see if you can get all your muscles to participate in the process. Not only will you find it easier, it will be less taxing on your tissues and you'll be far less likely to get hurt.

the challenge of complexity

The modern orientation towards functional movement also grows out of a heightened appreciation for the astounding level of complexity that we're now finding in the human body. In the old days of physical training, we imagined that the whole enterprise of training and treating the human body was pretty straightforward. It appeared that we could simply take an element-by-element approach; find out which parts of the system are weak and strengthen them with targeted exercises. As it turns out, things are far more complicated than we thought.

We get an appreciation for this complexity by looking at kinetic chains, the primary players in animal movement. At it's most simplistic level, a kinetic chain is merely a series of muscles that combine to produce a particular movement. The first muscle in the chain contracts, then the second and so on. Of course, the chain also includes elements such as tendons, ligaments and bones. These elements are coordinated and synchronized by an incredibly complex set of sensory and motor nerves. In this sense, the kinetic chain is a chain with a brain.

The first level of complexity has to do with the sequence of muscular contractions. When a kinetic chain goes into action to produce a movement, there are usually a lot of muscles involved, with many possible firing sequences. To get an efficient, skillful movement, it's essential that the muscles contract in the proper order. If you want to be strong, fast and functional, it's essential that you get the timing right.

For every movement there will always be an ideal sequence of contraction that will produce the best result. For example, if you're throwing a rock, you might want your legs to contract early to provide a base, then the abdominals to solidify your core, then the large muscles of the chest, followed by the finer muscles around the shoulder joint. If you get the sequence just right, the rock will fly fast and true. But if you've got the sequence wrong, it doesn't matter how strong the individual elements are. If you fire the muscles in your shoulder too early, for example, your throw will be weak, inaccurate or injurious.

This is why bodybuilding is such a poor method of athletic conditioning. The vast majority of the exercises are devoted to isolating individual links in the chain, while almost no time is devoted to practicing the sequence, timing, integration or orchestration of muscular contraction.

Sequence, by the way, is not only important for performance, it's also a vital component of injury-resistance and rehabilitation. Obviously, if you're trying to perform a vigorous movement without firing your muscles in the right sequence, you're going to over-load certain tissues and experience more fatigue and long-term wear and tear. Being strong in individual muscles is no defense; unless the elements are contracting in the proper sequence, your odds of injury are increased.

To make matters even more complex, there's also the fact that the muscles in a kinetic chain don't simply contract and relax in a binary, on-off fashion. Rather, there are overlaps in the duration and intensity of the contractions. Muscle 1 contracts, then muscle 2, but muscle 1 doesn't simply contract and then go limp. It may maintain a certain degree of contraction to add stability or provide a base for the rest of the chain. If you look at muscle-activity graphs recorded by kinesiologists, you will see a complex, overlapping series of curves, even for simple movements. Clearly, this is an extremely complicated study.

So, once again, we see the limits of isolation as a training method. Yes, you might increase the raw strength of individual muscles, but that's all you'll get. Unless you practice specifically for the movement you want, there is almost no chance that you'll get the proper sequence, timing or coordination that you're looking for.

When we look at the full complexity of kinetic chains, we begin to appreciate just how many things can go wrong with the system. Weakness might be the problem, but given the importance of nervous system circuitry, we might also say that the chain is only as strong as it's slowest link. Or to be more blunt, we might say that the chain is only as strong as it's dumbest link. Maybe the neurological connections to the muscular link aren't working at their best efficiency; the muscle itself is OK, but the wiring is down.

If the cybernetic, nervous system feedback loops aren't working right, there is no way that the chain can function properly, regardless of how strong the links are. If there's a deficiency in sensation or a timing error, the contractions in the chain may not come in the right order. And even if they do come in the right order, they might not come in the right intensity or sustain for the right duration. As you can see, there are millions of potential problems with kinetic chains, which is just one more reason to train them as whole units.

When we begin to appreciate the daunting level of complexity of the human body we are left with two basic choices for physical training. On the one hand, we can try to pick apart the individual elements and map out precisely how the nervous system and muscular system interact. If we're really diligent and smart, we may be able to come up with solutions and highly-targeted exercises. We might, for example, determine that a particular muscle in the chain is a little slow to contract. We then figure out an exercise that challenges this muscle to contract a little more vigorously. If we're really expert, we might be able to pull this off.

Or, we can simply train the body in a way that mimics that challenge we are trying to prepare for. In other words, we can train functionally. In this way, we simply bypass the challenge of complexity and orchestrate the myriad components into a single whole.

lessons from the imaging studies

Dramatic support for the functional orientation also comes from recent studies on musculoskeletal pain and injury. In days past, most of us have assumed that pain is the result of some structural defect in the body. Some tissue is cracked, fractured or torn, something is too long, too short, misaligned or twisted.

It makes sense to think that flaws in structure would lead to pain and other problems. Surely a short muscle, torn ligament or twisted spine could lead to pain. This belief has led physicians to seek out ever more sophisticated imaging technologies that would allow them to see the details of internal body structures. X-rays, MRIs, CT scans and bone scans held great promise in this quest. For the first time we could see the internal structure of the living body and we leapt to the assumption that it would now be a simple task to correct structural problems.

Once again, it turns out that things are a lot more complicated than we thought. A series of studies reported in the March 1998 *Sports Medicine Digest* suggests that our structuralist assumptions may have been misguided. In these studies, researchers took medical images of large numbers of "asymptomatic" people–individuals who reported being pain-free. What the studies revealed is that many people have "significant anatomical abnormalities that have no obvious clinical significance." In other words, it is now becoming clear that there are many people walking around with problems such as herniated spinal disks and torn rotator cuffs and yet have no pain and are fully functional.

These findings are immensely significant and will become pivotal in the future development of our medical, rehabilitation and fitness philosophies. They effectively demolish many of our cherished assumptions about how our bodies work and how they can be most effectively treated when something goes wrong. As the authors of the study put it,

> The medical establishment once hoped that sophisticated imaging tests would become primary screening tools that could identify pathology in need of treatment. The studies documenting asymptomatic abnormalities have firmly squelched this expectation. The notion that an MRI can reliably reveal the cause of pain is the beginning of a perilous thought process.

In other words, pictures don't and probably can't tell us everything. You could take an ultra-detailed, full-color moving picture of the inside of your shoulder joint and it still may not reveal why you're in pain. Structure, as it turns out, is only part of the body's story. Another way to describe this situation is to say that the correlation between structure and pain is relatively weak; some people have nearly perfect bodily structure and experience pain, other people have horrible structural defects and yet manage just fine.

Knowing the structure of your body through advanced imaging may be desirable, but it is far from sufficient. If your knee hurts, it's a good idea to have a specialist take a picture, but don't assume that this will yield a definitive answer. It may even lead you astray by showing you structural problems that are irrelevant to your condition. That ragged flap in your meniscus might be the cause of your knee pain, but maybe not.

The untold story here is the role of the nervous system, especially the way that it adapts to changes in the body's structure. In times of musculoskeletal distress, the nervous system attempts to work around pain. The locomotor system has lots of redundancy built into it; there are usually several combinations of nerves and muscles that can perform a movement. If a primary muscle is injured or somehow inhibited from performing its normal task, the competent nervous system simply re-routes the motor command to a secondary circuit and the job gets done, not as efficiently perhaps, but adequately nonetheless.

Looking at the human body from an evolutionary perspective, this ability to shift control from primary to secondary neuromuscular pathways makes perfect sense. In fact, it would be truly astonishing if the vertebrate nervous system did not include some provision for the re-routing of motor commands around sites of pain and weakness. If we lacked this ability our bodies would be super-fragile; we would never have made it out of Africa.

Of course, some people are better at re-routing nervous system signals than others. Some of us, typically the physically untrained, are stuck in a neuromuscular quagmire and are unable to move motor signals around pain and weakness. For these people, even minor injuries can be extremely problematic. On the other hand, people with rich physical experience–athletes, dancers, and actors–can do neuromuscular work-arounds with relative ease. After all, they've done it many times before. For these folks, even major injuries can be tolerated surprisingly well. Since they're experienced compensators, they simply shift the load onto healthy tissue and carry on.

Of course we would be fools to disregard structure entirely and we can be thankful that there are specialists out there who know the fine details of human structure. Anatomy will always be important, but as we begin to understand the nervous system in greater detail, we will begin to train people functionally. We will spend less time trying to see inside people's knees, shoulders, and ankles and more time teaching them how to move around inevitable structural defects.

functional orchestration

When we take a functional approach, we begin to think of our physical training as a sort of musical practice in which the component parts of the body come together to make harmonious, integrated music. Obviously, the ideal is to get the strings, the wind instruments and the percussion sections playing together. In contrast, the isolationist approach concentrates exclusively on individual elements of the body's orchestra. The string section may become super-strong, the wind instruments may become technically proficient and the percussionists may learn the most complex rhythms, but unless they actually spend time practicing together, the orchestra will never really make great music. Individually bulked-up elements don't necessarily add up to an integrated, harmonious whole.

Obviously, the individual elements have to be up to the basic task; some isolation training may be called for. If your string section is out to lunch, you won't make beautiful music. Each section of the orchestra has to be strong enough and skilled enough to play their parts. But the ultimate objective is always harmony. If the entire group–the whole body–practices together frequently, integration becomes far more likely.

You get what you play for

In one sense, exercise science is a highly complex, intricate, multi-layered discipline. Each system in the body is composed of millions of individual elements, interrelationships and feedback loops. We could easily spend a lifetime studying any one of them. The more we look at the body, the more intricacies are revealed.

If we look at it from another perspective however, exercise physiology really becomes quite simple. We can even go so far as to summarize the entire process in a single sentence. That is, the body makes extremely precise changes to meet the challenges placed upon it. Physiologists have coined a term to describe this process: the SAID principle. This awkward acronym stands for "Specific Adaptations to Imposed Demands." It is one of the most important principles of physical training; unfortunately, it is also one of the most commonly overlooked.

After decades of studying the effects of exercise, we now know that the body adapts with exquisite precision to the stresses that are imposed upon it. If you challenge your body to do a particular activity with some degree of regularity, it will attempt to make physiological changes to support future cases of that activity.

If you squat in the dirt and bang rocks together in an attempt to make stone tools, and do this regularly over the course of weeks and months, the tissues in your body will adapt specifically to meet the demands of this rock-banging movement challenge. The skin on your hands will thicken, the circulation in your legs and forearms will change, your nervous system activity will adapt to send faster and more precise signals and, if continued for long enough, even your bones will undergo a transformation, precisely proportional to the intensity and duration of your tool-making behavior. After a while, you'll be in good shape for making stone tools.

The lesson for modern fitness is clear: our bodies adapt precisely to the loads and demands that we place upon them. If you challenge your body to stand on a tight rope and juggle bowling pins and practice this movement with some frequency, your body will try to provide physiological support. If you challenge your body to swim underwater or sing in a clear voice, your body will attempt to modify its anatomy and physiology to make that possible. It will change muscle tissue, nervous system firing patterns, chemical and enzyme concentrations and hormone levels. The body is always at work, trying to detect patterns of physical challenge and build tissues that support future cases.

We see this everywhere: long-distance runners develop huge coronary arteries, swimmers develop an increased lung capacity, musicians develop extremely fine motor control. Skateboarders and snowboarders develop keen sensitivity to position and momentum. In the days before hiking boots, sherpas in Nepal developed thick callouses on their feet.

Incredibly, we also see the same thing in the fossil record. Fossilized skeletons of *Neanderthals* and early *Homo sapiens* reveal right-side humerus (upper arm) bones that are of significantly greater diameter than the left, a pattern that suggests powerful, regular movement of the right or dominant arm. This enlarged bone diameter is very similar to what we see in modern tennis players.

Every few years *Outside* magazine does a profile on the elite class of deep water divers and their preposterous feats of physiological endurance. These divers routinely dive hundreds of feet into the ocean and hold their breath for minutes at a time. Some of them even carry spear guns and hunt for big fish. Obviously, these individuals are extremely "fit," but you might not know it by looking at them. Sure, some of them have a barrel chest that tells of prodigious lung development. But this is only a small part of the physiological story. Besides their obvious pulmonary development, we can be sure that these divers also have developed extremely fine adaptations in their nervous systems as well as profound changes to their blood chemistry, things that are impossible for us to see by casual observation. All of these changes are specific to diving deep under water; they might be of some use in other activities, but this is not necessarily the case. It is the combination of adaptations that makes for performance.

In one sense, the human body is actually dumb and reactive. It conserves resources whenever possible and only modifies tissues as necessary to meet a cyclic, ongoing demand. (Which is actually pretty smart when you think about it.) From an evolutionary perspective, this SAID principle makes perfect sense. When the young animal is born, it has no idea what kind of conditions it will encounter. Environments are always changing. Temperatures may become hot or cold, food may become highly concentrated or widely dispersed, water may be abundant or scarce. The animal with a single, static set of physiological characteristics would be at a distinctive disadvantage compared to one that is more pliable and adaptable. Thus, natural selection has given us a body that is capable of an astonishing range of adaptive changes. It can modify its physiology to tolerate temperature extremes, dietary changes, changes in elevation and so on. Load up a body with some sort of challenge or stress and the body will adapt as precisely as it possibly can.

Remember, humans are habitat generalists; during the course of a lifetime, we may be called upon to traverse a wide variety of terrain. We might need to walk and hunt in the deep snow of polar regions, the sandy soils of arid deserts, the wet and muddy paths of rainforests, or the steep and rocky terrain of high mountains. Each of these terrain types demands a different kind of physiological adaptation. Walking in sand, for example, is a completely different challenge than walking over rocky hills; each uses different muscles with different nervous system patterns.

Scientific American described a good example of the SAID principle in it's *Men 1999* issue (see "The Mystery of Muscle"). As many amateur athletes know, muscle tissue in the human body consists of two basic types. "Slow," or Type 1 fibers convert raw materials to energy relatively slowly and are best suited for muscles that must contract with great frequency over long periods of time. Muscles of the back and legs are rich in these "slow" fibers. We also have "fast," or Type II fibers that are capable of more powerful contractions. These fibers are ideal for short bursts of powerful, hunting, fleeing and similar movements. To a certain extent, the distribution of these fibers is directed by our genetic code; some people simply have more "slow" fibers in their legs and thus make better distance runners. Nevertheless, this ratio will change in response to activity. A few years of concentrated strength training will stimulate production of "fast" twitch fibers, but if you switch to running marathons, you will actually replace many of the "fast" fibers with "slow" fibers that are better suited to the activity. In other words, you'll experience a specific adaptation to the demand that you imposed upon your body.

It's easy to see how this process would work in the ancestral environment. Suppose that your tribe spends a season in dry, hilly terrain. Maybe your hunting style requires short bursts of high-intensity movement; running up and down hills, for example. This activity stimulates a specific physiological adaptation; you produce more fast-twitch fibers. But now suppose that the climate changes or your tribe migrates and now you spend a couple of seasons on a broad, grassy plain. The only way to get food is to chase the herds over long, flat expanses. Now your activity stimulates another adaptation; you replace some of those fast-twitch fibers with more slow-twitch.

Of course, there's more to physiological adaptation than muscle tissue. Neurologist Harold Klawans put an especially juicy spin on the SAID principle in his book *Why Michael Couldn't Hit*. Jordan, as you may remember, retired from basketball in mid-career and took up baseball, where he floundered miserably. Klawans had predicted this outcome based on what he knew about the nature of the human nervous system. From a neurological perspective, hitting a moving baseball with a bat is a far different skill than throwing a basketball through a stationary hoop; each requires it's own particular set of nerve cell adaptations, it's own set of connections, it's own wiring.

When Jordan was in his youth, he challenged his nervous system to develop in a particular, highly specific way; he challenged certain sensory cells to send messages to his spinal cord and certain motor circuits to direct highly accurate, graded contractions in his muscles. His nervous system responded to these challenges with highly specific adaptations, especially growth of connections between nerve cells. These adaptations were of little use in hitting a fastball.

They were however, plenty strong enough to sustain one of the most impressive comeback performances in the history of sport.

twins in action

We can prove the SAID principle through a simple thought experiment. Take a pair of identical twins, raised in an identical environment. When they reach adulthood, put them on different cardiovascular training programs. Twin A goes to the pool for intensive, regular conditioning 4 times per week. Twin B runs trails 4 times each week. Match the programs for overall intensity and continue the program for a couple of months or so.

At this point, both of the twins will be healthier than before and both will have good cardiovascular capability. But now ask them to switch roles; send Twin A to the mountains and Twin B to the pool. The results are predictable. While each of the twins is likely to perform competently, there is no way that either could match the performance of his specifically trained brother; the swimmer will suffer on the trail runs and the runner will struggle in the pool. Both are healthy, but each has developed a set of highly specific physiological adaptations for his individual life.

velocity specific

The most fascinating thing about these physical adaptations are how incredibly specific they can be. One researcher took two groups of people and put them on a simple bench-press resistance program. He instructed one group to lift at a slow speed. The other group was to perform the same movement, but at a higher rate of speed. Both groups trained at the assigned speed and added weight to the bar when possible.

At the end of the study period, the researcher found that each group had made strength gains, but primarily at the speed at which they trained. In other words, the slow group got significantly stronger at slow movements, while the fast group got stronger at the fast movements. There was probably some overlap, but in general, the adaptations were specific to the imposed demands. The athletes got what they trained for.

This finding, by the way, invalidates claims made by some trainers that everyone must lift, move or run in a particular way. How could that be? There is no universal fitness formula. In fact, we would have to say that both the slow lifters and the fast lifters were "more fit" and healthier after the 6 weeks of training, but in completely different ways. If there was only one human environment or one set of physical challenges, then yes, we could say that there is a single best way to exercise. But there are thousands of possible fitness objectives and demands, thus, there are many ways to train.

cardiac adaptations

The more we study the human body, the more examples we see of the SAID principle in action. Consider this bit of research reported in the journal *Circulation,* 1999. The study found distinctive differences between the hearts of endurance-trained and strength-trained athletes. Or, to put it in the language of medical science, researchers found "divergent cardiac adaptations" in response to different types of exercise.

Using an electrocardiograph, researchers measured the wall thickness and internal diameter of the left ventricle of the heart, the chamber responsible for pushing blood out to the extremities. In strength-trained athletes, they found "significant wall thickening and modest changes in internal dimensions." This makes sense. If you're pushing big iron, you need to move blood to your tissues, but you don't need to move a large volume because the challenge is basically anaerobic. You're not relying on oxygen delivery to feed high numbers of muscular contractions, so your heart doesn't have to deliver much beyond baseline.

In endurance-trained athletes, researchers found a "pronounced increase in both wall thickness and internal diameter." Again, this makes sense. If you're running a marathon or riding a century, you need to move a lot of blood and you need to move it a long way, from your heart to the big muscles of your legs. Since you're now working aerobically, you depend on oxygen delivery and you're asking your heart to respond with greater volume.

The most interesting adaptation was in those athletes who pursued some sort of strength-endurance sport such as rowing or cycling. Here the researchers found the largest increases in wall thickness and internal diameter. In other words, the hearts of these athletes adapted to move big quantities of blood with power and authority. We can also assume that their coronary arteries grew in diameter as well, since the heart itself needs more blood to produce these powerful, high volume contractions.

This study suggests, by the way, that for individuals who are primarily interested in developing cardiac capacity and preventing heart disease, power-endurance events may be the best option. In other words, instead of just running a bunch of miles, we might be better off running middle-distance events or powerful intervals, sessions that demand the sustained application of strength. Ask your heart for both greater strength and volume and it's likely to deliver.

neurogenesis

When challenged, the body generates specific adaptations in all systems: muscular, endocrine, digestive, immune and so on. Fascinating new discoveries in the field of neuroscience now reveal that the nervous system also produces adaptations in the form of neuron death and growth (a process called neurogenesis).

For decades, researchers believed that humans are born with a fixed number of nerve cells and the new growth and reorganization is impossible. But recent work by Elizabeth Gould at Princeton University has shown that new neurons are produced in the brains of mammals, including primates. Gould showed that neurogenesis is most pronounced when the organism is exposed to a complex, stimulating environment. From what we already know about other physiological adaptations, it makes sense to assume that the growth of new neurons is not random. Rather, it will be specific to the challenges faced by the creature in question. If we challenge the organism to solve a puzzle, lift a weight or exploit a new food source, it will generate new neurons and neural connections in an attempt to make these behaviors possible. The body is always recreating itself.

professionals

Professional coaches and athletic trainers may not use the same terminology as we're using here, but in practice they pay close attention to the SAID principle. It's obvious—you don't train a basketball player the same way you train a powerlifter. You don't train a speed skater the same way you train a baseball player. You train for a sport by playing that sport; you prepare for a task by doing that task and closely-related variations.

Military trainers are also devoted to the principle of specificity. To be sure, the armed forces are notorious for administering blanketed programs of physical abuse and "character building," but this is generally inflicted on raw recruits and is intended more for psycho-social conditioning than authentic physical preparation. Once discipline and order is established in boot camp, the training becomes more sophisticated and specific to intended outcomes. Modern military trainers are devoted to this orientation. You don't train a fighter pilot by playing baseball; you train a fighter pilot in a simulator that mimics actual conditions as closely as possible.

no free lunch

The SAID principle tells us that there is absolutely no free lunch in physical conditioning. Some therapies and substances may support the body's return to physiological baseline after injury or illness, but there is only one way to go above that level and that is challenge, in other words, movement, exertion, striving and sweat. The language of the body is challenge and response. If tissue is not challenged, it will not adapt. It has always been this way. With the exception of placebo effects and similar mental influences, no one has ever increased his or her strength, endurance or agility by any method other than by exercising those very qualities. No skill was ever developed except through the act of striving for that skill.

Old-school coaches had a crude understanding of the SAID principle and trained their athletes by the harsh dictum "No pain, no gain." The idea was simple: force the body to adapt by overloading it with some kind of excess demand—push the body and it will respond. Unfortunately, this crude understanding led to crude application, frequent injury and widespread stupidity. It also had a negative side effect in the way that it came to influence popular exercise practices. Reluctant exercisers, when exposed to the threat of a mandatory pain regimen, are likely to turn around and head back to the couch. Or, they'll abuse themselves indiscriminately under the belief that pain itself is the necessary element. Now, as our understanding of exercise becomes more sophisticated, we begin to see that it's not pain that stimulates our bodies, but challenge. Now we say, "no challenge, no adaptation." In other words, if you don't push your comfort zone a little, your body isn't going to pay attention. It's not the pain that makes the difference, it's the push.

setting personal objectives

The goal of physical training is to stimulate to body to produce the physiological adaptations that you're looking for. To do this, you've got to impose the right demands, with the right intensity at the right frequency. That's all there is to it. You set the training agenda and your body will do it's best to generate appropriate adaptations. At this point, it becomes obvious that we need to give some serious thought to our personal training objectives. What is it that we are trying to do with our bodies? What kind of adaptations do we want?

Dedicated athletes know their objectives; they want to execute their movement specialty well enough to win a championship. But for the average exerciser, the situation is not nearly so clear. Most people say that the want to "get in shape" and let it go at that. But this is a horribly vague objective that gives us no guidance whatsoever. And if our objectives are vague, it's highly unlikely that we'll make any progress. Instead, we need to narrow our focus and identify those activities that we really want to pursue. What exactly is it that you want to do with your body in the next couple of years? In five years? In twenty?

The temptation here is to fall back on cosmetic objectives and say for example, "I want to lose ten pounds." That puts the cart before the horse. A better starting point is to think about what kind of functional performance you're going to be looking for in the future. For example, my functional objectives for my 70th birthday go like this: "I want to be able to hike long distances without fatigue, up to 10 miles per day. I want to be able to carry a pack that includes enough overnight gear for a three-day outing. I want to be able to go off trail onto rough terrain without spraining my ankles or losing my balance. I want to be able to cross creeks and snowfields without stumbling. I'd like to be able to set up camp, cook dinner and scramble up a nearby ridge to watch the sunset. Then I'd like to be able to hike onward the next day to my next camp and so on."

In any case, it's essential to be highly specific in setting your objectives. It's not enough to just say "I want to be able to swim." You've got to say how far, how long, what conditions, and any other detail that might be relevant to you. The more detailed you can make your objectives, the more precisely you can target your training and the better results you will achieve.

So, instead of listening to a "fitness expert" tell you how many sets, reps, miles or pounds you need in your workout, decide exactly what it is you want your body to be capable of and challenge yourself to do exactly that. Make a list. Do you want more endurance? More power? More speed? Decide what capabilities you want and train specifically for those qualities.

Many people say that they want to be able to work in the garden, for example. This is a good functional goal, but it needs detail. Gardening actually involves a wide variety of sub-tasks such as squatting, digging, pruning and lifting. Do you want to do long hours of pruning or planting? Carry sacks of fertilizer? Dig weeds? Stand on a ladder? Dig post holes? If you think about these tasks now, you can create exercises that stimulate the adaptations that you're after. In fact, you could create an entire exercise program based entirely on the objective of developing garden fitness.

Another functional objective I often hear is "I want to be able to play with my grandchildren." This is great functional objective that brings us full circle to the origins of human movement. But "play" is not specific; we've got to break it down to it's basic elements. If you think about what's involved in children's play, you'll see that it involves short bursts of acceleration and deceleration, a variety of gaits such as skipping and hopping, throwing and catching, grappling, chasing and evasion. If you wanted to get really serious about this, you could break it down further and train for particular durations and intensities of each, but of course, if you trained that hard, it would cease to be play.

In any case, these kinds of lists will set your training agenda and help you design your program to be specific to the results you want. If you want speed, train for speed. If you want power, train for power. If you want balance and grace, train for balance and grace. Design your program to suit your life, not the theoretical conditions established in a laboratory or the mind of a gym rat. Train for the way you want to live.

The joys of therapeutic trauma

In the old days, people imagined that exercise was directly and unequivocally good for the body. "Do a workout," they said. "It'll make you stronger, faster and healthier and you'll feel better too." We assumed that there was something special about vigorous movement that stimulated good health.

This, as it turns out, is only true in a roundabout way. The actual facts are surprising and counter-intuitive. What we are now discovering is that vigorous exercise is injurious to tissue, sometimes extremely so. During strenuous exercise, metabolic waste accumulates in tissues, cell membranes burst and blood vessels suffer micro-trauma. Muscle fibers tear and scar tissue rips apart. A flood of free radicals wreaks havoc on all tissues. There is no longer any doubt on this score. For even the most superbly conditioned athlete, exercise *is* injury.

This makes exercise sound unpleasant and in the short term it certainly can be; occasional soreness is an inevable part of the fitness game. The good news is that the payoff comes later in the form of physiological rebound, a process that exercise scientists and coaches call "super-compensation." Incredibly, the body recognizes the injury, cleans up the mess and builds new tissue that is superior to the old, at least in terms of that particular challenge. This process works particularly well if these exercise-inflicted injuries follow a fairly regular pattern of oscillation. Over the course of months and years, the body becomes superbly adapted to the challenges it has experienced. This process is at work in all forms of vigorous movement, from the intense strength training of power-lifters to the long-distance endurance training of runners and bikers.

When administered in an intelligent, oscillating pattern, we would be correct to describe exercise as "therapeutic trauma." Professional coaches and trainers recognize this clearly and are highly adept at inflicting precise forms of injury on their athletes. They do not push indiscriminately nor do they inflict injury for the sake of injury. Instead, they study patterns of stress and compensation and inflict injuries that will closely mimic the strains that their athletes will encounter in action. If the micro-injuries on the practice field are precise in intensity and form, and if the challenges oscillate with periods of deep rest and rejuvenation, athlete's bodies will compensate quickly and effectively.

When thinking about exercise, we naturally tend to focus on changes in the cardiovascular and muscular systems of the body. But we have to assume that a similar process is at work with the nervous system as well. When we push hard in an intensely challenging exercise or skill session, we're pumping gobs of neurotransmitters across synapses. If we push really hard, we're probably going to exhaust some nerve cells and cause some kind of microscopic injury. We might blow some cell membranes or deplete their ability to manufacture fresh transmitters. We then experience this nervous system injury as lethargy, weakness or awkwardness in the days following the big effort. When the supercompensation comes a few days later, we feel agile, skillful and powerful.

Keep in mind that not just any injury will stimulate a compensation for increased strength, endurance or higher performance. Just because it hurts doesn't make it therapeutic. Pain and injury in and of themselves do not cause performance gains. Just because you're suffering on the track or at the gym does not mean that you're making progress. It is only precise, intelligent and well-patterned injury that causes supercompensation and progress. In all cases, the dose makes the medicine. What we need in training is an optimal level of injury. Injury that falls above or below this optimal level will be either ineffective or counter-productive.

As our understanding of physiology grows, our understanding of exercise becomes more paradoxical and interesting. Physical therapists and trainers like to tell clients that "exercise is medicine," but it might be more accurate to say that "injury is medicine." It's not so much that we need regular exercise to remain healthy; what we need is regular injury. Of course, this notion isn't going to gain

much popularity, but it does make for some interesting thought experiments.

Here we would do well to make a distinction between exercise for health and exercise for high performance. Each demands its own level of therapeutic trauma, its own degree of self-inflicted injury. If all we want is to maintain a modest level of well-being, we don't need to inflict a high degree of punishment on ourselves. Periodic low-level assaults on the muscular and cardiovascular systems are probably enough to keep the body reasonably pliable, capable and happy. If we inflict a little microscopic injury, we'll enjoy a lot of gain.

But if we want to excel at a sport or high-intensity movement specialty, there can be no avoiding the issue; we're going to have to hurt ourselves in an intelligent fashion. We'll need to inflict significant damage to the right tissues and we'll need to do it often. Naturally, this puts us squarely up against an obvious risk; the trauma may go too far. There's a very fine line between high-intensity traumatic exercise and a career-ending injury. It's easy to miscalculate and wind up with the worst possible combination: a lot of pain and no gain. This is the line that all professional athletes have to walk.

Naturally, we can go too far with this orientation towards "therapeutic trauma." If a little self-inflicted injury is a good thing, we might reason, then a whole lot of self-inflicted injury must be better. But only a fool goes to the extreme with this principle. There are limits to how much injury the body can tolerate and compensate for. If the exercise-inflicted injuries are too deep or come too frequently, the body will be unable to compensate. Tissue damage will accumulate and all your gains will be lost or reversed. At this level, exercise becomes an act of futility or just plain self-abuse.

The other fresh insight that comes with this orientation is that, if you are exercising with any kind of regularity, you will often be in a low-level state of injury, at least in a microscopic sense. This also means that you will frequently be in a state of rehabilitation as well. Injury is not something that just comes along every now and then, after an awkward fall or a particularly strenuous game; rather, it is a near-certainty. And by the same token, rehabilitation is not something that you'll only do after a major traumatic event; it is something that you'll be doing every day.

As athletes and coaches become more sophisticated in their approach to exercise, they look for ways to limit the therapeutic trauma or injury to the desired physiological targets. If you are looking for particular adaptations, keep the injury in that zone and don't allow it to carry over into other areas. For example, if you're training for a big bicycle race, you want focus your self-inflicted injury precisely on those tissues that contribute to speed and endurance on the bike. If you inflict excess collateral damage by training outside your primary movement challenge, you'll simply add to your injury load and draw precious healing resources away from where you want them.

Obviously, therapeutic injury must be applied in an atmosphere of safety and professionalism, but within these bounds, there is nothing wrong with a direct and adversarial approach. Be sure to emphasize the yin side of recovery to match the yang side of exercise-induced injury. There is a place for benevolent injury in our repertoires.

As functional exercisers, we should injure ourselves and we ought to do it well. The whole point of the enterprise is to cause microscopic tissue damage of just the right degree with just the right frequency. If we can provide the right kind of tissue injury, the body will respond with superbly appropriate adaptations.

As we learn more about the nature of exercise, it becomes obvious that the trick is to inflict these therapeutic injuries on ourselves in a sophisticated, intelligent pattern. Haphazard, random infliction of exercise induced injury will not do us much good at all. Instead, we have to present the body with a pattern that it can understand.

Animal kinetics

There are countless possible ways to move the human body. With hundreds of muscles and millions of nerve cell pathways, the combinations of speed, power and agility we can produce are essentially unlimited. Given this vast range of possibility, it's easy to get lost in the complexity as we try to select effective exercises and training methods. We can attempt to pick apart the individual elements involved–the muscles and neural circuits that control them–but such an enterprise could span lifetimes.

Fortunately, there appears to be a common pattern within all this diversity, a single unifying quality of animal movement that we can put to good use. Biomechanical specialists now recognize an oscillating curve that is common to most animal movement–an alternating, rebounding pattern that is not unlike the bouncing of a ball or the stretch and rebound of a bungee cord. This movement pattern is the foundation of physical education and is essential to success in movement, injury prevention, rehabilitation and performance.

terminology

In it's simplest form, the basic pattern of animal movement consists of two phases and a transition. In the first phase, the muscles, tendons, and ligaments are taken into a stretch, either by gravity, momentum, or by the contraction of opposing muscles. This is followed by a transition as the movement reverses direction. In the second part of the cycle, muscle fibers contract and an action is produced. There is a clearly identifiable feel to this kind of quality movement. It bounces. It compresses and expands. It winds up and delivers. It dances.

The basic phases of this movement cycle are actually pretty easy to understand. Unfortunately, biomechanical specialists have come up with all kinds of conflicting terminology to describe them. For example, the initial phase has been called a "pre-motion," an "eccentric contraction," "pronation," "force reduction," "shock absorbtion" and "storage of potential energy." The second phase has been described as "acceleration," "supination," "force production," "concentric contraction" and "energy release." Martial artists even describe these movement phases with the terms "yin" and "yang." It's no wonder that we're confused.

Fortunately, we can ignore the terminology for the time being and concentrate on the basic character of the movement. One way to study this is to imagine that your body is rigged up, not with mysterious muscle tissue, but with garden variety bungee cords. (This is actually not too far off the mark; muscle tissue does have an elastic quality that is not unlike shock cord.) Now imagine what it would feel like to move. First stretch and then rebound. Pre-motion then motion. Pronation then supination. Force reduction then force production. Yin then yang. In case you've forgotten, this is what it feels like to be a child; the young body has an elastic quality that bounces.

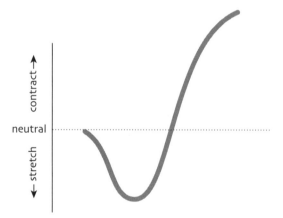

The prototypical animal movement is represented by this curve, depicting the amplitude of movement over time. What we see is a pre-motion, a transition and a movement. Together, these phases add up to an elastic, oscillating, rebounding movement that we see in all high-level dance and athletics. Accomplished physical artists

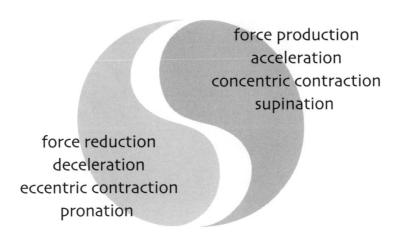

force production
acceleration
concentric contraction
supination

force reduction
deceleration
eccentric contraction
pronation

learn to modify this quality of movement in many variations by making it shallower or deeper, faster or slower, but the essential sense of physical rebound is always there.

the biomechanics of fly fishing

The prototypical movement of the human body closely resembles the dynamics of the fisherman's fly rod. Like a human limb, the fly rod is a resilient, elastic structure; when disturbed, it has a strong tendency to return to its original shape. The fly rod also shows a gradient of flexibility and elasticity along its length; it is stiff at the base and flexible at the tip. This is similar to what we see in the human torso and extremities; the biggest muscles attach to a powerful base (the hips, pelvis and lumbar spine) and progressively become more flexible and delicate towards the hands and feet.

The most intriguing similarities come in movement. Watch the way the fly rod behaves during the casting cycle. When we look at the action, we see that the rod cycles through the back cast and then reverses direction to the front cast. In the back cast, the weight and momentum of the fishing line pull the elastic fibers of the rod into a stretch, which then rebound to pull the line forward in harmony with the contraction in the caster's arm. So, we see that the fly rod goes through a loading phase in which the elastic fibers come under stretch, then into an active power phase or forward cast.

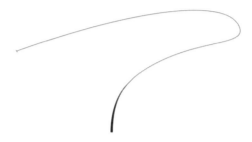

During the back cast, kinetic energy is stored within the fibers of the rod which is then released during the forward cast. This is analogous to what happens to a human limb that moves through an active range of motion. The fly rod pronates, then supinates. Force is reduced, then produced. In fact, in term of their kinetics, the fibers of the fly rod and the human arm are doing almost precisely the same thing.

improving performance

If you want to improve your physical performance, it is essential that you gain some physical understanding of the basic movement. You can study this for yourself by going back to that grade school standard, the standing broad jump. First try it from a dead static starting position. Get down into a crouch, then pause for a couple of seconds to let all the movement dissipate; let your legs relax. Now jump as far as you can from a dead start. If you like numbers, record the result, or at least make note of the sensation. Now try the jump again with a fully dynamic movement. Drop down into your crouch and rebound out with a fast, smooth transition. If you're like most people, you'll go significantly further. Plus, you'll be able to feel the difference. If you practice the transition, you'll find that you can smooth it out, adjust the timing and improve the final result.

You can feel the same effect in other basic movements. Try to touch the basketball rim from a dead crouch, then with a dynamic motion. Try throwing a ball from a dead position, then with a complete wind-up. No matter what movement you're trying to perfect, study the depth of the pre-motion and the timing of the transition. If you can perfect these phases, the rest of the movement should take care of itself.

the nervous system component

There is more to the playful primal movement than the simple elasticity of muscle tissues; our bodies are more than sticks and bungee cords after all. The transition between phases of movement is always mediated by the nervous system. Several things need to happen for an effective transition. First, the position sensors in our ankles, knees and hips must be fast, accurate and sufficiently loud to inform the central nervous system of where limbs are in space. If you don't know exactly where your arms and legs are or how fast you're moving, it is unlikely that you will be able to manage the transition. Second, the motor nerves must be sufficiently fast and concentrated enough to change the direction of the movement. If you can't recruit enough motor units for a fast and powerful active contraction, the transition will be slow. This spells poor performance and injury.

The goal here is to build skill. Specifically, the idea is to work on the timing, to synchronize your contraction to come precisely at that moment when the natural elasticity in your tissue is at its peak. In a way, the skill is similar to learning how to synchronize your pull when working on a playground swing set. Pull too early and you waste the natural swing. Pull too late and your effort is wasted.

hitting the brakes

The most underrated and least-practiced part of the basic animal movement is the pre-motion or wind-up that we see on the left side of the curve. Typically, we are focused on the ultimate outcome of the movement and so we tend to emphasize the more obvious, late-stage action; the right side of the curve. But it's the quality of the pre-motion that makes it all possible. If your wind up has the right shape, depth and timing, it will lead to a smooth transition and a powerful and agile final expression.

A key component skill here is the ability to decelerate. Clearly, you can't carry too much speed in the wind-up phase because you won't be able to turn it around into an complete movement. So, you're going to have to manage the motion and dampen it as you approach the transition point. In other words, if you want to move fast or powerfully, you've got to learn to manage movement; you need to learn how to decelerate.

The muscular dynamics of the human body are similar in certain respects to the behavior of the automobile. In a car, we have two separate components for acceleration and deceleration; an engine to speed up and a set of brakes to slow down. The human body also has the means to accelerate and decelerate, but the difference is that both of these functions are performed by a single component: muscle. (Or, more properly, neuromuscle.) In other words, muscles can function as either accelerators or as brakes. It just depends on how you use them.

When we think about acceleration and deceleration of the human body, we're likely to think of gross, whole body acceleration such as we see in the 100 meter sprint. But from the point of view of the physical therapist or movement specialist, the most interesting thing is that acceleration and deceleration events take place, not just for the body as a whole, but across every joint in the body, often in tiny, super-fast alternations.

For example, if you run a 100 meter sprint, you'll obviously want to accelerate down the track and then decelerate after you cross the finish line. But even during the course of the race itself, you'll be performing thousands of microscopic, highly precise acts of acceleration and deceleration in your effort to run as fast as possible. In fact, skillful acceleration and deceleration of individual body segments is essential to producing full-body speed. In this sense, great sprinters are not only skilled at acceleration, they are also highly skilled at deceleration.

It helps to think about the movement of individual body components here. For example, consider the leg as it swings forward during the sprint. It's moving fast—you can't simply throw it out in front and let it go at that. You'll want to control the length of your stride and the placement of your foot when it strikes the ground;

accurate foot placement is important. This means that you'll want to decelerate the motion with your hamstrings; during this phase of movement, your hamstrings are the brakes.

Of course, as your body passes over the foot, you want to transmit power through the leg. So now your hamstrings become accelerators. Thus, as you run the 100 meters, your hamstrings perform a high-intensity, rapid oscillation: accelerate, brake, accelerate, brake and so on. The same goes for all the muscles of your legs, torso and even your arms. The complexity of this act is astonishing; the level of neuromuscular synchronization in even a poor runner is a monstrously sophisticated computational task.

The ability to decelerate is vital, not just in running, but in every dynamic skill activity. It's not enough to introduce motion; that motion must be controlled. The point guard running towards the basket must manage a monstrously complex act of deceleration as he approaches the hoop. The figure skater must continuously dampen forces that threaten to spin out of control. The boxer who throws a jab must decelerate the stroke before it extends too far.

In terms of raw physical education, deceleration is the more difficult skill to learn. Young athletes can often produce good acceleration of individual body segments, but since their braking skills are poor, they lack control. Flailing limbs, wild pitches and sloppy execution are often the result of poorly developed braking skills. This is why physical educators and coaches should emphasize control before power and grace before speed.

It's also important to remember that injury-resistance depends in large measure on our ability to apply the muscular brakes with speed, precision and effectiveness. If you can't decelerate your body movements smoothly and precisely, your joints will suffer more microtrauma, and in some cases nasty macrotrauma as well. Thus, one of the most important skills in physical education is deceleration. We can invent games and exercises with this specific goal in mind, or we can simply pay more attention to physical grace and control. If you're moving gracefully, you're certain to be decelerating skillfully as well.

Walking the walk

First, there was the foot.

Marvin Harris
Our Kind

O ne of the primary objectives in any physical training program should be to build a better biped. Walking is our primary movement pattern and the ultimate source of functional performance in all our daily activities and sport. Locomotor efficiency is fundamental to almost everything that we do. It doesn't matter whether your personal objective is proficiency in gardening, basketball or blue-collar construction. If you don't walk well, it's unlikely that you'll excel at any athletic or functional movement.

Walking is routinely dismissed by serious athletes and amateurs, who consider it far too elemental to devote any attention to. Rarely do we hear anyone brag about being a good walker. But as it turns out, walking is an incredibly complex, composite skill that demands a high level of coordination. In fact, when we study the intricacies of human locomotion from a physiological point of view, we are struck with wonder that anyone can do it at all.

born to walk

When asked to describe the defining characteristics of *Homo sapiens*, most of us talk about language, tool use, intelligence, opposable thumbs and consciousness. These are certainly valid candidates, but in terms of our actual history, they were actually late developments. The original and most important adaptation in human evolution was upright walking–bipedalism. Walking came millions of years before language, tool use and culture. As paleoanthropologist Donald Johanson put it, "Bipedalism is what made us human."

Naturally, anthropologists are constantly revising their estimates for the original appearance of bipedal locomotion in hominids. Many of these estimates place the earliest bipedalism at 4 to 5 million years ago. A recent find in Central Africa may push that date back to 6 or 7 million years ago.

Of course, if you really want a date range to remember, a good figure is 3 to 4 million years ago. This is the time of the fabulous set of footprints discovered by Mary Leaky at Laetoli, Tanzania. At this site, a small band of hominids walked across an area of soft dirt which was then covered by a layer of volcanic ash, preserving the prints in a pristine state.

This is also the time of Lucy, the famous, nearly-complete *australopithecus* find that showed dramatic skeletal evidence of bipedal structure. These are not the original cases of bipedalism, but they are certainly some of the most spectacular evidence that we've got.

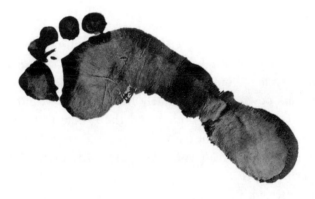

For our hominid ancestors, walking was the key to staying alive. As the climate of East Africa dried and cooled, the forests began to thin out. As they did, primate food supplies became increasingly dispersed. No longer could your tribe simply amble across a small clearing to a nearby fruit tree and spend the afternoon snacking; now you'd have to hike to the other side of an immense valley. Of course, you might get lucky along the way. As vigilant opportunists, your tribe might happen across a fresh kill abandoned by a carnivore, but in general, food was scattered. If you wanted to eat, you'd have to put in some miles.

There were other reasons to walk as well. Once our ancestors learned how to make stone tools (perhaps 2.5 million years ago), they had to secure the raw materials. You can't make a good stone tool with just any rock however, and the good ones weren't always handy around camp. The hominids used many widely-dispersed stones including green lava, white quartzite, chert (a type of silica), quartz, granite gneiss and pink feldspar. These rocks were probably spewed across the landscape by volcanic explosions. Working in and around Olduvai Gorge, Mary Leaky concluded that early humans must have either traded or traveled to secure materials from many miles away. There was no overnight FedEx rock delivery. Clearly, there must have been a lot of walking and carrying involved. If you wanted some quartzite to make a hand axe, you had to go and get it.

know your phases

Given the absolutely crucial importance of gait, we need to do a quick review of the basic elements, the primary phases of the walking cycle. Biomechanical professionals have broken these movements down to an absolutely freakish degree, but fortunately for us, we only need to understand the fundamental movements. Once you understand the basic elements of these phases, you'll be in a good position to create your own games and exercises to enhance your performance.

Let's start with swing phase, that period of time when your leg is swinging free to take your next step (Officially, this is the time between "toe-off" and "heel strike.") Imagine that your right leg is swinging free into your next step. Throughout this phase, you're standing on your left leg and your center of gravity is now unsupported; the only thing that keeps you from falling to the right are the quick and highly coordinated contractions of the muscles on your left side, particularly those on the left side of your hip.

The timing of these contractions must be just right. That is, the muscles on your left hip must come into contraction precisely when your right foot is leaving the ground. They must then relax just as your right heel contacts the ground at the end of swing phase. If the contraction comes in early or late, or with insufficient intensity, you'll have an inefficient gait, higher impact forces and greater chance of fatigue and injury. A tiny flaw in timing, repeated over the tens of thousands of steps you might take in a typical day could add up to substantial fatigue or tissue inflammation.

Once your heel touches the ground, you enter the stance phase, that period from "heel strike" to "toe off." At this point, the challenge becomes one of weight acceptance, shock absorption and force production. Necessary elements include speed, strength and timing. You must immediately absorb shock and stabilize the leg as the body passes over the foot. Biomechanically, this is no easy task; the impact force can be up to several times body weight. This impact must be absorbed by a precarious stilt-like structure that is inherently unstable.

Not only that, but this shock absorption must be extremely fast; as your leg accepts your body weight, the muscles must fire in a fraction of a second. The time between "heel strike" and "toe-off" will naturally vary with your speed and style, but in any case, it's not very long. The contraction and stabilization of the leg must come into play during that interval. If it's early or late, the leg will not be sufficiently stabilized and stresses will fall on to other non-muscular tissues such as ligaments and joints.

pronation and supination

Biomechanical specialists analyze human gait in minute detail, joint by joint, muscle by muscle. But for the average exerciser, this level of analysis can get overwhelming pretty fast; we don't need to know all of the subtle dynamics of the ankle joint to be better walkers, for example. A simpler way to understand it is to think of bipedal locomotion in the more general terms known as pronation and supination.

In the pronation phase, the leg absorbs shock by rotating slightly inward at the ankle, knee and hip. This is a normal motion that takes place with every step. When the shock is fully absorbed at mid stance, the leg should begin to rotate back laterally towards its original position as it powers the forward movement. As one leg is pronating, the other is supinating and vice versa. The movements are complementary.

Unfortunately, some people have come to the conclusion that pronation is a pathological disorder that condemns them to a life of sub-standard running performance and inevitable injury. Actually, pronation is a normal, essential part of bipedal locomotion. Over-pronation might be a problem, especially if the arch of your foot collapses or if your leg rotates too far inward or fails to return back to its supinated position. In cases like these, a physical therapist may be able to help you reduce the level of pronation with strengthening exercises or orthotic inserts. Nevertheless, it's important to remember that pronation is not a disease. It's a normal component of gait, subject to occasional distortions.

we are monopeds

In high-level athletic and physical therapy programs, coaches often spend long periods of time working with people in the one-footed or monoped position. Curious beginners often wonder about this practice. We aren't monopeds, they point out—we're bipeds.

It is true that we are bipedal primates, but contrary to appearances, we actually do spend an astonishing amount of time on one foot. In normal human gait, stance phase and swing phase alternate in a complementary fashion; when one leg is swinging free from back to front, the other leg is supporting the body. All of the time that you are swinging one leg forward, you are in fact standing on one foot.

According to Jacquelin Perry, author of *Gait Analysis*, single limb support accounts for 80% of the total gait cycle. In other words, you are supported by either one leg or the other for 80% of the time you are walking. The remaining 20% consists of double leg stance at the beginning and end of each phase. When you're running, the situation is even more pronounced; full speed running is conducted entirely on one leg or the other. In other words, if you run a marathon, you do 13 miles on one leg, 13 on the other.

If you look at your waking hours and assume that you walk for much of each day, as a hunter-gatherer would, you will realize that we actually do spend a huge percentage of our time on one foot. The increments are small, but they add up. If you spend 6 hours hiking for example, you will have spent about 4 hours and 50 minutes on one foot or the other and only about 1 hour and ten minutes standing on both feet simultaneously. (And even this is with one foot forward, one foot back.) Even when we're standing still, we usually stand with most of our weight on one foot or the other. So, in this sense, we *are* monopeds. And, we could go so far as to say that the objective of functional training is to "build a better monoped."

This is why functional movement coaches spend a lot of time training their athletes and patients on one foot. By building balance and useful strength in one leg at a time, stance phase becomes more stable and gait improves. This has a prehabilitative effect on your ankles, knees, and hips. Plus, it's can be a lot of fun; there are dozens of games that can enhance your monoped skills.

biped training: improving your locomotion

There are many ways to improve your locomotor performance. Obviously, you're going to have to get out and walk and that's going to take some time. And sorry, you don't get to count the walking you do between the car and the video store. No, I'm talking about putting in some genuine mileage with your hands free and your mind engaged on the task at hand. Here are some possible variations:

simple endurance walk

This one is an act of imagination in which we strive for maximum efficiency. Imagine that there's been some sort of crisis event on the grassland; maybe your tribe has been split up by a storm or separated by predators. Maybe a big grass fire has swept across the bush and now you need to make it to the next valley before nightfall. In any case, you have a long walk ahead of you and you'll need to save every shred of energy. With this predicament in mind, make your movement super-smooth. Eliminate any excess motion or tension and let your legs swing in long, loose strides. Concentrate on balance, sensitivity and economy of motion. Make your gait sustainable.

hunted gatherer walk

Here's another act of imagination. Suppose that you find yourself alone in unfamiliar region of scattered trees, bushes and intermittent clearings. Light is falling and you suspect that there's predator activity in the area. Now take that image into the present: that's not a house cat behind that car, it's a leopard. That dog's not on a leash; he's part of a hungry pack. Danger comes from above as big cats lurk in your neighbor's trees. You may have to break into a full speed run at any moment, there's just no telling. Walk deliberately with maximum balance and agility.

stealth walk

Think of this one as a sort of tai chi walking exercise, an opportunity for concentrated study of locomotion. By moving with super-slow deliberation, you can attend to any of the individual components or sub-movements. For example, you can study the way your center of gravity shifts from left to right, the way your feet meet the floor, the way your knees absorb your weight or the way your abdominals stabilize your hips and torso. Alternately, you can work with a variety of fantasy images. Pretend that you're a ninja sneaking into the emperor's castle. Pretend that you're crossing a frozen lake with thin ice. Or that you're trying to make it down the hallway at night without waking a sleeping dog. In any case, sustain the exercise for several minutes at the very least; you'll be amazed at how challenging it is.

creative running

When faced with the possibility of running for exercise, many of us quickly find other things to do. The activity sounds plain boring: put one foot in front of the other, then repeat for about a million repetitions. In fact, this is exactly how many people go about it, enduring long, monotonous "sleep runs" in which the only variations are occasional dog attacks or swerving cars. When we do it this way, running *is* boring.

But there's nothing to say that you can't have fun and turn your run into a highly productive and therapeutic dance. Start by breaking up your run with variations on basic locomotion. Try skipping for awhile or running backwards. (Skipping is not for sissies!) Try cross-stepping with a lateral run. Change your speed with bursts of acceleration and deceleration. Now try lengthening your stride by just a little bit. Throw in a few quick and graceful 360's every few yards. Slalom around imaginary obstacles. High-step over imaginary rocks and logs. Pretend there's a minefield on your route. Run on your toes. Try super slow running with giant steps. Then try running as if you're being chased by a carnivore.

Or, stick with your standard gait and pace, but shift your attention to different areas of your body. Go a few hundred yards, paying close attention to the way your feet hit the ground. Go another hundred, and feel the way your arms drive your legs. Go another hundred and concentrate entirely on your abdominals and the way they support your movement. Go another hundred and think about nothing but the quality of your breathing. Now smooth the whole thing out and pretend that you're so efficient and smooth that you could run for 3 days without stopping. And finally, when you're getting back to your car or your house, accelerate into a glorious, silky smooth sprint as if there's no tomorrow. Who says running is boring?

By the way, if you do all these gait variations that I've listed here, you're going to attract attention. People on their porches and in their cars will point their fingers at you and question your sanity. But that's OK. Remember, you are the normal human animal, doing a normal animal thing. If the sedentary people in your neighborhood find your behavior amusing or entertaining, that's all well and good. After all, they probably need some action in their lives. Don't let their opinions stop you.

intervals

Most of us associate running with aerobic endurance and overlook the fact that running is also very much a skill event. There is a strong nervous system component here and there are millions of possible adjustments that we can make to improve our locomotor efficiency. But learning these kinds of adjustments demands a high level of concentration and attention, something that is extremely difficult to sustain over the course of a typical 5 mile slog. Even if your attention to detail is strong, your mind is bound to wander.

A good solution here is to do intervals. By breaking up your run into smaller blocks of effort, you can apply a much higher level of concentration to the subtleties of your movement. For example, choose an interval distance that works for you–maybe a lap around the high school track, maybe just 100 yards. As you run this distance, focus as intensely as possible on what you're doing. Pay maximum attention to the quality of your gait; make it as smooth and powerful as you possibly can. Then walk an easy interval until you're sufficiently recovered, then repeat, again applying your maximum possible concentration. By oscillating between focused concentration and relaxation, you'll develop your locomotion skills to a much higher level than would be possible in a longer effort. And, you'll still reap some of the vascular rewards that come with a sustained run; interval training is really good for your heart.

Fast interval running offers another possible advantage: lower impact forces. This sounds backwards, but not if you think of the basic mechanics involved. When you run, your movement can be described with two vectors, one goes up, the other goes forward. If you're running in place, your vertical component is 100% and your forward motion is zero. If you're running really fast, the forward vector dominates and your vertical movement is just enough to help you stay upright. The greater the vertical component, the higher the impact forces. In other words, slow running may actually be more demanding than sprinting.

Another bonus of interval training is that you can make it social. Get together with your pals and do the intervals together. Push hard on the runs, then walk back to the starting point together. As you walk and rest between efforts, you can catch up on all the news. This is easier and more interesting than trying chat while you're in the midst of a five mile run.

strength training

For modern athletic trainers and coaches, it is becoming increasingly clear that we can improve our bipedal performance with intelligent strength training. The biomechanics are complex, to be sure, and there is plenty of controversy about the details, but consensus is emerging on a few key ideas.

First, core body strength and intelligence is vital. If your abdominals are weak or slow, you'll have poor control over your hips and pelvis as well as poor coordination between upper and lower body. Thus, any kind of abdominal work that you do is likely to improve your walking and running skills.

Second, hip extension is fundamental. Your butt and hamstrings power your stride. A weak butt not only means poor extension, it also means that less rotational control of your legs, which in turn places more stress on your knees. Thus, squats, lunges and step-up are likely to make you a better walker and runner. Uphill walking and stadium stairs will also put some power into your hip extensors.

going barefoot

If you've ever explored the cult of high-performance running, you know that shoes and orthotics are an obsession. Manufacturers, consultants, podiatrists and physical therapists have built a vast industry around the biomechanics of the foot and ankle. No matter your gait profile, foot shape or event, there's a shoe or insert that will—it is claimed—work for you. The promise is alluring; if you can add a half of a degree of ankle support with a custom orthotic, you might run just a little bit faster in your next competition and you might even get over that pain in your heel.

The study of biomechanics can get pretty interesting, but all of this obsessive attention to shoe design and modification completely misses the fact that the natural state of the human foot is shoeless. We have run and walked barefoot for the vast majority of our existence. Shoes are a recent invention, a novelty.

This might just be a minor point of issue, were it not for the fundamental fact that people walk and run differently when barefoot. The biomechanics are completely different. You can prove this for yourself by going to the park and running barefoot over a variety of surfaces—grass, dirt and gravel for example. Of course, this probably strikes you as ludicrous. Maybe you haven't run barefoot in years or decades, and now you're worried about stepping on something sharp or yucky. That's exactly the point. When you run barefoot, you'll run lightly and with lots of attention, precisely the way humans have run for most of our history. You'll be on your toes more than usual and you'll be paying far more attention to what you're doing. In other words, your gait will be entirely different.

This suggests that footwear, even if technically perfect, can never be a total solution for performance enhancement or injury rehabilitation. It also suggests that, if you want to make your training truly natural and holistic, you'll do some occasional barefoot running or walking. Now obviously, there are some practical considerations here. Foot injuries can be nasty and you'll want to exercise some intelligence in choosing conditions. Nevertheless, you may discover that including some barefoot walking and running into your exercise sessions can be extremely revealing and possibly therapeutic. At the very least, you'll get a broader diversity of movement and you'll enjoy a big increase in sensory contact with the ground—qualities that are valuable for any body. And if you're lucky, you might just find a primal gait pattern that helps you work around pain or injury. We desperately need more research in this area, but we can be sure that barefoot locomotion holds great promise.

rough it

Trainers and coaches who work with human locomotion are beginning to discover that rough, uneven surfaces are essential for effective neuromuscular training. This orientation is supported by recent work of Boston University bioengineer James Collins. Collins discovered that adding "noise" to the sensory nervous system aids the detection of weak neurological signals. Specifically, he found that the noisy signal generated by a vibrating footplate pushed weak nervous system signals above a detection threshold and thus improved his subject's balance. Collins built a mechanical set of insoles to introduce noise to the sensory neurons of subject's feet. In experiments, Collins found that his subject's showed significantly less postural sway when using the device than when standing on solid ground.

Sensory neurons in our ankles, knees and hips are threshold-based and these thresholds tend to increase with injury, age and lack of use. Reduced sensory ability, naturally, leads to poor function, inefficient movement, falls and injuries. If you live in a world of smooth surfaces, your nervous system won't receive much stimulation. Smooth, level floors and sidewalks just aren't "noisy" enough to keep your sensory-motor nervous system operating at peak efficiency.

Collins' invention promises to improve balance and locomotor efficiency among elderly patients, but we could achieve a similar result by encouraging people to simply go hiking on uneven ground. This would be particularly effective when using thin-soled trail shoes instead of hiking boots. Every little rock, every uneven root, every slippery patch of moss introduces a little bit of noise that boosts the detection of tactile signals. Rough terrain wakes up the sensory nervous system and makes your body smarter.

poles are for tents

If you've done much hiking in the last few years, you may have noticed a pronounced increase in the number of people using ski poles while they hike. Where I live, in the Pacific Northwest, this trend has become so popular that it is now becoming rare to see people hiking without poles.

At first glance, hiking with ski poles makes a certain amount of sense. By turning yourself from a biped into a triped or quadruped, you can increase your stability and possibly avoid falls and ankle sprains. And, if you apply some upper-body power to the poles, you might be able to increase your efficiency and thus delay fatigue.

On a given day, you may do well with the poles, but in the long run, the benefits become drawbacks. As you learn to depend on your poles for balance and stability, your innate balance circuits begin to slack off. They aren't being challenged to such a great degree, so they don't respond. If you use the poles regularly for a few years, you may find that your balance and agility on the trail actually declines. And now, you're really going to need the poles.

A better approach is to go without poles unless you really need them for genuinely treacherous terrain. Do your regular hiking as a biped; challenge your balance circuits to do their job. Keep your ankles, knees and hips awake by challenging them to adjust and support your torso on rocky ground. Then, when the going gets really dicey, get out the poles.

mind-body

When we set about trying to improve the quality of our loco-motion, we run into a curious relationship between what we're thinking and how we're moving. Véronique Dubost, a researcher at Saint Etienne University in France, asked people to perform tasks involving speaking or thinking while walking. She discovered that, not only did the walkers slow down as they concentrated, they also walked with shorter strides. Apparently, we share attention between mental and motor tasks, and in some cases, cognitive tasks can draw resources away from physical movement.

This research result suggests that there may actually be something to the time-honored jock stereotype. If you're really concentrating on physical performance and sensation, you'll have slightly fewer neural resources to spend on cognitive tasks. By the same token, if you spend most of your time devoting resources to cognitive prob-lem solving, you'll have slightly reduced physical performance. This is not to say that either is superior or preferable, simply that these individuals show a different distribution of attention.

We can also apply this kind of speculation to our ancestral hunter gatherers striding across the plain. Obviously, their minds were free from mental calculation; they hadn't gotten around to inventing arithmetic. And they probably didn't engage in a whole lot of in-ternal conversation either. The vast majority of their psychophysical resources went straight into locomotion and sensory acuity. Free from distraction, they must have been spectacularly powerful walk-ers.

In contrast, the modern mind is saturated with cognitive prob-lems, challenges, puzzles and dilemmas. We are calculating almost constantly, trying to solve the conundrums of relationships, income, mortgages, taxes and making a living. It is no wonder that we are in such poor physical condition; our hyper-active brains are constantly drawing resources away from our bodies.

We can use this understanding to inform our training programs. That is, if you're serious about walking well and improving your per-formance, you might do better if you leave your troubles and your mental calculations at home. Do your problem solving when you're driving or taking a shower. Or, if you do use walking as a time to solve problems, don't expect to gain as much physical benefit along the way. This is another reason why we can't count errand walking as part of our locomotion totals. If you're walking from the car to the mall, you're probably engrossed in your objective–getting to the movie on time, finding an address or remembering to pick up a grocery item. The last thing you're paying attention to is the quality of your gait.

Social walking has similar limitations. There is obvious value to strolling with your friends; you'll enjoy the conversation and build your relationships. But if you're deep in conversation, you're simply not going to improve your locomotion very much. If you want to get serious about building the functional strength and endurance in your legs, you may want to go solo or train with someone who knows when to be quiet.

We don't know much about the effect of listening to music while walking or running, but I suspect that we'll see similar effects. Clearly, music stimulates a different part of the brain than arithmetic and verbal problems, but it's not hard to imagine that there would be some sharing of psychophysical resources going on here. Portable music is extremely popular, but it may actually be a drawback for exercisers. Yes, you may derive motivation from your favorite licks, but music can also divide your attention. When your mind is occupied by music, you're not going to be paying attention to the subtle, vital sensations coming from your feet, ankles, knees and hips. And if you need tunes to get you moving, maybe you'd be better off finding a more enjoyable kind of movement.

Core considerations

These days, abdominals are a hot topic. Fitness bookshelves are packed with books on abdominal training and all of them offer some promise of "taut," "etched," "ripped" and even "legend-ary" abs. One book promises to "Banish Your Belly" while another claims that it will help you "Lose Your Gut." Inevitably, these books present a cover photo of a lean, well-developed torso, playing right into the cosmetic and weight loss motivations that drive so many of us. Some of these books make a bit of a concession to function, posture and back support, but in the main, the emphasis is consistently on appearance.

When we take a functional orientation on the other hand, we're primarily interested in how well we move and here we find that the abdominals play an essential role. For all animal athletes, powerful and efficient movement originates in the core of the body. The abdominals are, or should be, the primary links in the kinetic chain. Whether you are performing a tennis serve, a golf swing, a 100 meter sprint, or lifting a sheet of plywood out of your truck, the abs should provide a stable base from which the extremities can move.

the abs in prehistory

All primates have abdominal muscles, of course, and they are pretty much the same from species to species: a wrap-around, 3-dimensional corset that protects the internal organs and provides both stability and movement for the musculoskeletal system. Fossil remains of hominids don't tell us much about the state of our ancestral abs, but we can safely assume that they were nearly identical to our own; standard-issue, primate abdominals.

Throughout prehistory, the abdominals gave our hominid ancestors a solid foundation for a diversity of movement. Acting together with other muscles of the hips and shoulders, their abdominals solidified and unified the hominid torso and provided a base for locomotion as well as hunting and gathering movements. They created stability in the spine and the pelvis and helped to coordinate movement between the upper and lower body.

It's important to understand the fact that abdominals make an essential contribution to effective bipedal locomotion. If we were to observe a bipedal runner from a bird's eye perspective, we'd see that his hips and shoulders are always rotating in opposite directions, a twist-untwist movement of the spine that helps power the movement. If the abs fail to contract fast enough or if the contractions are poorly synchronized, two things will happen. First, locomotion will be slow, awkward and inefficient. Second, these rotary stresses will be absorbed by deeper structures such as the small muscles, ligaments and joint capsules of the lumbar spine. This means microtrauma and possible injury. Clearly, the abdominals are absolutely vital to graceful and sustainable walking and running. Without functional abdominals, we never would have made it out of the Pleistocene.

anatomy

If we really want to understand the abs and how to train them, we need to review a bit of anatomy. The popular image of the abdominals is that they lie exclusively on the front of the body, in a single strip that runs vertically, from sternum to pubis. This is the much-adored "six-pack," the *rectus abdominus*.

This, however, is only one layer of the abdominal wall, and is not even the most important one. Underneath that vertical strip are 3 more layers that run at a variety of angles, wrapping around the torso, encircling the abdominal cavity and attaching to the ribs, the pelvis and the lumbar spine. Two oblique layers consist of diagonal fibers that cross one another in opposite directions. The deepest layer, the *transversus abdominus*, is entirely invisible from the surface, but is interesting because it's fibers run horizontally. When these fibers contract, they squeeze the abdomen in the same fashion as a belt.

The criss-cross, diagonal nature of these muscle layers implies a tremendous diversity of possible movements. You can twist and flex, twist and extend, rotate, tilt your pelvis or turn your rib cage. The combinations are endless; the abdominals are capable of initiating just about any kind of movement/stability combination that we can think of. In turn, this capability implies that there are a lot of ways to train the abs as well.

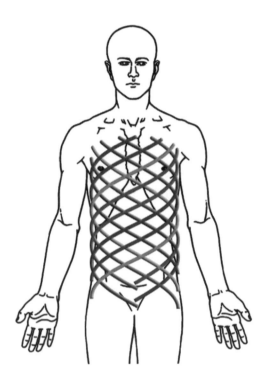

Another way to think about the anatomy of the abdominals is to remember that the human torso is divided into two primary compartments or cavities. The upper compartment contains the heart and the lungs; this is the thoracic cavity. The lower compartment—the abdominal cavity—contains the digestive organs: the liver, spleen and intestines. Between the two compartments is the diaphragm, a large, dome-shaped muscle that drives our breath.

To simplify it, think of your abdominal cavity as a box whose sides are made up largely of muscle. The roof of the box is your diaphragm and the floor is your pelvic bowl. In the front is the vertical strip of muscle, the legendary 6-pack. The sides of the box are composed of the oblique abdominal muscles, diagonal fibers that wrap all the way around the sides of the box and attach to a sheet of fascia that connects to the lumbar spine.

Acting together, these muscles create stability and control a wide range of movement, just as we'd expect, but they also have a deeper, less obvious effect; they raise the pressure inside the abdominal cavity. This so-called intra-abdominal pressure is created by the combined contractions of the transverse abdominals and the diaphragm. This creates a non-compressible bubble in the center of the trunk which provides substantial spinal support and may help to protect the lumbar spine against injury. Many modern physical therapists and coaches now advocate abdominal training as a important element in maintaining back health.

training

These days we take it as a given that we've got to lay on the floor to do our abdominal conditioning. Typically, we are told to do crunches and related exercises in the supine position. From the degree of conviction with which these kinds of exercises are promoted, we might guess that humans have been doing this kind of abdominal training for centuries if not millennia. But that's not the case at all. My guess is that over the vast course of human history, from Lucy to Jim Thorpe, not one of our hominid ancestors laid on the ground to crank out sets of crunches.

Since the abdominals are composed of fibers that run in many overlapping directions and since they connect all around your torso, it is absurd to think that there is one single movement or method to train them. In fact, there are thousands of possible movements that challenge the abdominal fibers. If all you do is crunches, you'll have a few strong crunch fibers and little else.

And not only that, single-plane exercises such as crunches or pelvic tilts are simply inadequate to train the whole system anyway. A better approach is to emphasize diagonal, multi-plane motions. The point of the enterprise is to get many abdominal fibers to participate in creating intra-abdominal pressure; the more participation, the better.

Practice engaging your abdominals in the position of function; that is, standing up, walking and lifting. It does little good to have strong abs only when you're lying down. How do your abs work when you're actually living? You must know how to make them work in all positions, especially standing. Practice picking things up with full abdominal contraction.

integration

Ultimately, we want to train the abs as part of a complete musculoskeletal system. We want to work not just individual muscles, but long kinetic chains that run from torso to extremity. And, we want to do it in a position that mimics actual, real-world challenges that we're likely to face. In general, this means getting up off the floor and doing some authentic, functional movement.

Some exercisers will balk at the suggestion that we can train the abs in a standing position, but this is precisely what today's professional trainers and coaches are doing in clinics all across the country. Specifically, we try to get the torso to act as a strong, integrated link between the lower and upper body. We can train for this quality with whole-body movements, especially diagonal movements with the medicine ball, stretch cords and pulley machines.

Training in this integrated fashion will remind you, for better or worse, of manual labor. Shoveling snow, chopping wood and digging holes all require functional participation by the abdominals in the upright, bipedal position. If you enjoy this kind of labor, you can kill two birds with one stroke; concentrate on abdominal participation while you work. Not only will this improve your overall efficiency and delay fatigue, it will also give your core a good workout. Of course, if manual labor isn't your favorite activity, you can substitute a medicine ball and make a game out of it.

woodchops

There are a couple of simple patterns that you can adopt instantly. The diagonal slash or snow shovel movement, also known as the "wood chop," is extremely valuable. This is a diagonal stroke that moves from high to low or low to high. You can use a medicine ball, a dumbbell, a stretch cord or a pulley machine for resistance.

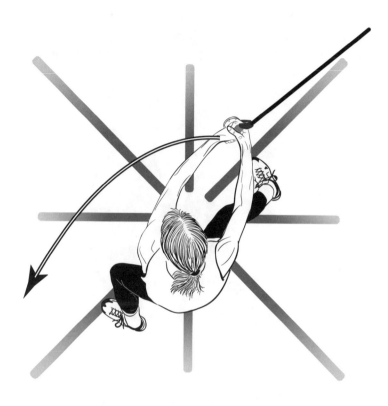

Stand with a wide base of support and proud posture, then move with authority. Pay particular attention to your hips and abdominals. Keep your arms and shoulders relaxed, with a strong central core.

figure eights

The most versatile of the functional abdominal movements is the figure eight. The beauty of this form is that you can generate dozens of variations that will challenge your core in a functional position, thereby integrating your abdominals with the rest of your body.

The basic movement is easy. Grab a medicine ball and swing it in a vertical circle on the left side of your body. Cross your center line in front of your navel, then circle on the right. Repeat in a continuous motion. A medicine ball is the most fun, but you can also do the movement with a dumbbell or a weight plate. You can also use two smaller med balls, one in each hand.

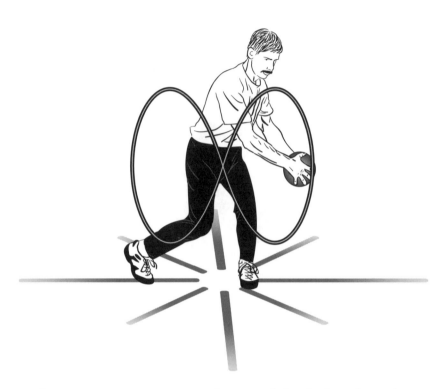

In any case, concentrate on using your abdominals and your butt. As you warm to the movement, begin to play with variations. Big movements will challenge your balance, smaller movements concentrate the effect deeper into your core. Slower movements will challenge your control, fast movements will drive the contraction home. Try stance variations as well: square to the front, lunge position, one foot and so on. Get low and make your hips do the work. If you're really ambitious, use a wobble board.

The other payoff here is that the variations on the figure eight will tie into lots of other functional and athletic movements: throwing, lifting, carrying, squatting. If you like martial art, you'll find dozens of blocks and strikes within the figure eight.

isolation

The ultimate goal in abdominal training is to build a stable core and to integrate your torso with your extremities as you train them to work together as a whole. Ultimately, you'll want to work the long kinetic chains that cross the hips and shoulders as well as the abs. In other words, you're looking to make your training holistic.

But for many people, the abs are so atrophied from disuse that they need the additional stimulation that comes with isolation; they need a wake-up call. In this case, it makes sense to get into the supine position, lying on the floor. This way we can put additional loads directly onto the abs which will wake them up and ultimately bring them into harmony with the rest of the musculoskeletal system.

You can crunch if you like, but you'll have more fun with a med ball. Lay on the floor, and hold the ball straight up above your chest. Pin your low back to the floor by squeezing your abs, then start moving with authority. Since your abdominal fibers run in all directions, you can move in whatever direction you like. Start with circles, both directions. Then do some slashing diagonal movements. Then some left-rights. And finally, a few thrusts straight up. If you've got a partner handy, they can hold up their hands as targets and heckle you for the best possible effort.

running and sprinting as ab training

We know that the abdominals play a vital role in human locomotion. Think about what's required during a sprint. Biomechanically, your goal is to produce maximum acceleration from what is essentially a stack of bones. You need stability, and most of all you need synchronization of the components. The abs are a major player here because they must transmit force between the upper and lower body. If the abs aren't working, you won't be able to stabilize the structure sufficiently to apply the power. Just imagine a bicycle with a really soft, spongy frame–such a device will be slow and dangerous.

In fact, it makes sense to speak of sprinting as a form of abdominal training in its own right. Try a series of short sprints. Make a conscious, highly intentional effort to tighten your abs, then take off running. Maintain the abdominal contraction as you run and try to intensify it as you accelerate. Notice how your torso now forms a solid, integrated anchor for your extremities. After 50 or a 100 yards, slack off and walk back to the starting point. Repeat often, and do it uphill if you can manage it.

all abs, all the time

The condition of our core muscles is so important to overall fitness that in a way, it becomes difficult to make a case for doing anything else but abdominal training. That's right, we could just forget the isolation exercises we typically do for our arms and legs. Forget squats, bench press, curls and rows. Just concentrate on the abs and nothing else. In fact, we could even devise a program devoted to nothing else but abdominal exercises: "All abs, all the time."

This is nowhere near as crazy as it sounds. But to make it work, we'd need to take a broad view of abdominal training. That is, you've got to look for the many ways to involve your torso in functional, standing positions. If you practice your movements with sufficient attention, walking, running and sprinting can be practiced as abdominal exercises. Then you can add squats and lunges, medicine ball work and basic martial art movements, all of which can be abdominally intensive. So there's really lots of diversity here.

The problem here is that this is fairly advanced training. Yes, you can train your abdominals effectively with walking, running and woodchopping movements, but only if you've got enough athletic experience to feel your abs in action. Many people's abdominals have gone so long without stimulation that they are essentially comatose. These individuals are less likely to benefit from these kinds of exercises. Instead, their abs need a concentrated wake-up call, typically in the form of supine isolation: crunches, medball circles, sit twists and the like. Then, once the nervous system has gotten back on line, they can stand back up and start into some functional movements.

Pipes and pumps

As our understanding of physiology grows more complete, it becomes increasingly obvious that this thing we call health has something to do with water. Some people have described the body as "a hairy bag of water," which is not too far off the mark. Obviously, we have a lot of water in our arteries, veins and capillaries, but we also have a lot of moisture between cells and within cells.

The thing that we're beginning to understand is that this moisture needs to be kept in circulation. Fluid turnover is essential to all metabolic processes. If the body's water stagnates, all sorts of physiological mischief can occur. It's more than just a matter of moving blood through arteries, veins and capillaries however; we need to move moisture deep within the body, all the way to the furthest reaches of the circulatory system. Some of this moisture can move passively along chemical and pressure gradients, but if you really want to keep fluids flowing through tissues, you've got to pump it actively.

If asked to name the primary pumping mechanism in the human body, most people would name the heart. This makes sense. After all, this four-chambered unit is an incredibly sophisticated marvel of efficiency. It pushes fluid for decades and, except for occasional hardening and narrowing of the coronary arteries, it performs almost without flaw.

Nevertheless, the heart is only one of the pumps in the mammalian body. We often overlook what I call the "musculoskeletal pump." Just as each contraction of the heart chamber moves fluid, so does each contraction of skeletal muscle. A contracted muscle becomes denser and exerts pressure on its vessels, thus squeezing blood and lymph down the pipe. In this sense, every muscle in the body is a pump. The larger muscles hold and pump an impressive quantity of blood—so much in fact that some trainers have even called the quadriceps (the big muscles on the front of the upper leg) "the body's second heart."

Alert readers will probably see where I am going with this. We all know what happens when someone suffers a heart failure. When coronary arteries close down, less blood reaches the heart muscle. If these arteries become fully blocked, a part of the heart muscle actually dies. Now imagine what happens if the musculoskeletal pump stops working. Or to put it another way, imagine what happens if you stop moving. At this point, your body is running without one of its primary pumps and fluid flow to and from your tissues drops dramatically. The effect won't be as immediate or dramatic as a heart failure, but over the course of a few decades, it will be just as pronounced and over time, just as fatal.

Losing your musculoskeletal pump is almost as catastrophic to your health as losing your heart pump. If your heart fails, you're going to notice it right away as your tissues cry out for fresh oxygen. If your musculoskeletal pump fails, the effects will be less dramatic in the short term, but equally damaging over the following months and years.

If you are in the midst of a long-term relationship with your couch, you can be sure that fluids aren't moving effectively through your body. In fact, since you aren't pumping, your body is on its way to becoming a virtual swamp. Your tissues may be getting superficial amounts of oxygen and you may be excreting a minimal level of metabolic waste, but that's about it. Cells at the furthest reach of your circulatory system are simultaneously starving and suffocating, regardless of how much you're eating and drinking. And all those expensive supplements you're taking? They may be dissolving in your digestive tract, but they're not getting pumped out to the regions where they can do you any good. You're lucky if they make it to your bladder.

The health benefits of exercise act on many levels. We've all heard about how regular movement maintains muscle tone, reduces stress and maintains bone density. But it may just be that the primary reason that exercise is so powerfully therapeutic is simply because it moves our metabolic juices. With this understanding, we can offer a new definition of therapeutic exercise: the act of pumping fluids through the body with alternating muscular contractions. In fact, we could even drop the word "exercise" altogether. Let's just say that we're going out to the track, the gym or the pool to do some muscular pumping.

It would be fun to create an exercise program based entirely on the objective of pumping fluid through the body. To be completely hip, let's call it "somatic hydrology." Just imagine how it might work. First, in order to move the most fluid, you'd want to involve the major muscles. The small muscles of your forearms won't pump much fluid, but the big movers such as your quads, glutes and hamstrings will really move the juice. Your butt in particular is a great pump. This means that we'd look for movements like squats and lunges and step-ups on the box. Running stadium stairs is a particularly pumpy exercise. Hiking uphill is another.

Second, we'd look for a rhythmic movements that oscillate between strong contraction and relaxation. Sustained stretches do not move fluid nearly as effectively as rhythmic movements. Just imagine that you're trying to squeeze the water out of a flexible tube; a constant pressure or constant stretch won't do it. You have to alternate the effort. This is why dance and dance-like movements are highly therapeutic; rhythmic undulations are not only fun, they're also good for us.

Third, we look for movements of large amplitude, those that cycle through a big range of movement. Obviously, a deep movement will pump more fluid than a shallow one. Walking with long, deep strides will move more water than a shuffle, doing a set of deep squats will move more fluid than a set of shallow movements.

Fourth, we look for an activity that you can sustain for a fairly long duration. A one-rep powerlift won't move much juice, no matter how much weight you have on the bar. Better if we can maintain the pumping for a few minutes or a few hours.

Of course, if you combine these three characteristics—major muscles, large-amplitude movement and long duration activity—you're talking about some serious sweat. Try running stadium stairs for a solid 30 minutes or hiking continuous uphill for an hour or more. If you're really into moving fluid, this is what it takes.

If you're rehabilitating after an injury, it is particularly important to move fluid. Tissues that are in the process of healing are extremely active; they require greater amounts of nutrition, oxygen, and glucose and they also generate more metabolic waste. Thus, in rehab we look for pumping movements that are low-resistance but highly repetitive. Instead of going right back to the weights, do lots of passive motion with the injured body part. Lots of easy, pain-free cycles can help nourish injured tissues.

warming up

Closely related to the idea of fluid movement is the idea of "warming up" before exercise. These days, the warm-up is dogma; most trainers tell us that we absolutely must warm up and that if we fail to do it we will suffer severe physical consequences. This advice has now become so reflexive that some trainers now advocate warming up before doing *any* kind of movement. Taken to the extreme, we might now assume that we have to warm up before warming up.

And yet, in spite of these claims, the value of warming up has not been backed up by any decent real-world research. Some people appear to need it, others don't. Post-race interviews with marathon runners have revealed no consistent pattern of injury that relates to warm-ups. Many NBA stars spend hours of pre-game preparation and are sweating buckets before the national anthem. Charles Barkley, in contrast, would put on his uniform, shoot a couple of jump shots and declare himself ready to go. Then he'd go out and put in a hall-of-fame performance. At best, our information about the practical value of warming up remains inconclusive.

If we look at warm ups in the context of hunter-gatherer evolution, we get mixed messages. On the one hand, we can assume our hominid ancestors probably slept late when possible and lounged in the sun before venturing off on their daily expedition. Naturally, they would do easy movement before pushing themselves; walking before running, for example. You don't just open your eyes, leap up, and start running after game. Obviously, if you're living in an uninhibited state of nature, you'll do some yawning, easy stretching and general movement before you get physically ambitious.

On the other hand, physical challenges on the grassland were fundamentally unpredictable. Carnivores could appear at any time and the hunter-gatherer might have to move fast and powerfully "off the couch." Thus, for total hominid functionality, we would need to be capable of diverse movements; warm up when possible, but know how to move from a cold start.

The same holds true for any mammal in a state of nature. The average dog can go from a stone-cold sleep to hot, mad feline pursuit in the blink of an eye. Sure, he might chase that cat even more effectively if he had performed a warm-up, but such an idea totally misses the point: mammalian muscle tissue is fully capable of cold-start movement. It may not be the ideal way to move, but it is not necessarily dangerous either. If cold-start movement was as dangerous as everyone says it is, mammals in the wild would consistently be crippled.

Of course, we need to remember that modern people are living in what is essentially a chronic state of stasis that is entirely different from our original experience. In the context of modern physical experience, many people are so far removed from regular movement that a warm-up becomes more essential. When a person has been "on the couch" for years or decades, cold-start movement probably is dangerous; in this context the warm-up becomes more important, even essential.

thixotropy

When pondering the objective of a "warm-up," most people assume that the idea is to get limber, flexible and well, warm. To be more specific, what we are really looking for is something called *thixotropy*. This term is used in the field of material science to describe the behavior of gel-like substances that become liquefied when mechanically agitated. The connective tissue in the musculoskeletal system is one of these gels. It's solid when undisturbed, liquid when manipulated. Sometimes these gels are called "fluid crystals."

When we look at it this way, we see that our fitness objective is not just to produce warm tissue. Rather, the idea is to produce liquefied tissue. Liquefied tissue allows for the easy flow of cellular fuels and wastes and at the same time it offers reduced resistance to muscular contractions.

The key to achieving thixotropy is not heat, nor is it the circulation of blood. Rather, it is mechanical agitation. In other words, movement. Gross body movements produce the desired result, not outside air temperature. This is why going into a sauna does not really constitute a warm up. In fact, you can actually produce some good thixotropy by shoveling snow in cold weather.

One common misconception is that stretching is the same thing as a warm up. Actually, these are two different things that happen to overlap slightly. Stretching can be valuable, but it doesn't deliver the necessary contractions that promote fluid movement and complete exercise readiness. True, stretching does offer some mechanical action and thus creates some degree of thixotropy. But if that's all you do, you'll miss some essential elements. If all you do is stretch, you won't warm the vascular system; your arteries and capillaries will remain in their cold, inelastic state. Thus, it might make sense to use stretching as a supplement to a warm-up, but never as a substitute.

If you want your warm up to be complete, you'll want to liquefy, not just your muscles, but the tissues of your vascular system, especially the major arteries that supply blood to your muscles. Remember, major arteries are wrapped with several layers of tissue, including smooth muscle. In their "cold" state, these vessels can only expand so far and are thus limited in how much fluid they can deliver. But if we can generate some thixotropy of the vessel walls, we can greatly expand our fluid carrying capacity. The way to do this, of course, is with some kind of vigorous, vascularly demanding movement, especially large amplitude pumping of the big muscles of the legs. As these muscles demand more oxygen and blood, they'll call on the arteries to soften and expand. If you oscillate your intensity–large amplitude squats and lunges alternating with short rests for example–your circulation will soon become pliable and ready for more intense action.

An often overlooked aspect of warm-up is the nervous system. Most of us concentrate our attention on muscles and ranges of motion, but we tend to forget the control system. But the nervous system, like any other system in the body, becomes more efficient with a preparatory phase. Every musician knows this to be true. Yes, the concert pianist wants the muscles in his fingers to be "warm" and he wants his capillaries dilated so that they'll carry fluid to and from the tissues. He might even soak his hands in warm water before the concert. But what he really wants is nervous system readiness. He wants his tactile, sensory nerve cells to be primed to carry messages from his hands to his brain and he wants his motor nerves to be ready to carry the integrated messages back to the muscles of his forearms and fingers. Without nervous system preparation, even the warmest muscles won't make music.

functionality

We assume that warm-ups are absolutely vital, and we use them prior to our workouts, but how does this correlate to the actual demands of our daily lives? It seems to me that if we are training for our actual lives, that we ought to examine what we actually do and train accordingly. I don't know about you, but there are thousands of times in my life when I need to move my body efficiently and powerfully without a warm-up. I don't warm up before I clean out the garage, put out the trash or move furniture around. And I won't be able to warm up before defending myself against an assailant on the street.

Instead of creating an artificial workout paradise, the superior course would be to train specifically for situations that we will actually encounter. Does the activity you're training for allow for a warm-up? If so, practice with the warm-up. But if the activity doesn't allow for it, practice from a cold start. Learn to move efficiently and powerfully "off the couch." Your tissues may not be at their optimal fluid best, but that's just the way things go. Work with what you've got. Learn to move your body under any conditions.

This is not to say that warming up does not have potential advantages. If your main concern is squeezing the maximum possible performance from your tissue and your nervous system, you really do want to be warm. If you're doing elite level athletics, the warm-up is an absolute necessity. If you're training for the Olympics, every hundredth of a second counts, so you want to stack the physiological deck in your favor. And, if you're trying to rehabilitate yourself after an injury, you also want to stack the physiological deck in your favor by coaxing your tissues into a fluid and pliable state. Complete thixotropy is your first goal; liquefy the tissue, then do your rehabilitative movements.

Wiring for health and performance

When we think of physical fitness, most of us think of muscle and fat; if we've got strong, lean muscles, people say that we're "in good shape." But while lean muscle is certainly an important part of the picture, it's only one element. Muscles themselves are actually pretty dumb. More important are the control circuits that tell the muscles what to do. Ultimately, our success or failure as good animals depends in large measure on our ability to harness the full capability of our nervous systems. A quick review is in order.

The human nervous system is composed of billions of cells called neurons. These range in size from microscopic blips of protoplasm to motor neurons as long as a human limb. Each neuron connects with at least one or as many as thousands of its neighbors. These sites of connection are called synapses; these junctions have excitatory or inhibitory effect on neighboring cells. These cells work together to form information processing circuits similar to but far more sophisticated than the average computer. The purpose of the nervous system is to integrate and coordinate the activities of all the other systems of the body; this is the master system.

they're all skill events

As our understanding and appreciation for the nervous system has grown, we are beginning to realize that we need to rewrite our descriptions of our favorite athletic events. According to popular belief, sporting events fall into a handful of basic categories: aerobic, anaerobic and mixed. Sports such as the marathon and long-distance bicycle racing are called "endurance events" while sports such as discus throwing and power lifting are called "strength events." Intermediate forms such as football and basketball tend to get classified as "mixed" or "strength-endurance." Finally, we tend to pigeon hole events such as archery as "skill events," those that don't demand much in the way of strength or endurance, but are nonetheless difficult and impressive. Casual observers of athletics assume that all events fit into one of these categories or the other.

But from what we now know about human physiology and the pivotal role of the nervous system, we can now say with confidence that *all* movement challenges are "skill events." It doesn't matter whether you're trying to row across the Pacific or lift a Volkswagen, you'll succeed or fail in large measure by the performance of your nervous system. Athleticism is always about skill.

Yes, some sports place conspicuous demands on the cardiovascular system or the muscular system, but even here we find powerful nervous system influence. The experienced runner who pushes hard over long distances is not just drawing on cardiovascular resources; his nervous system is actively involved throughout the event. Not only does it orchestrate fine adjustments in biomechanics, shifting his gait pattern and delaying fatigue, it also stimulates the production of essential hormones and neurotransmitters, stimulating some organs while inhibiting others. And in the so-called strength events, big muscles aren't enough; the champion is the one who can "recruit" the greatest number of muscle fibers. In this sense, strength is skill.

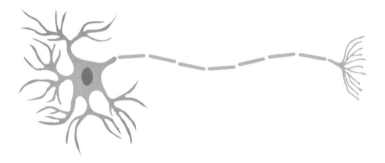

smart body, dumb body

When we think look at the role of the nervous system and the way that it is distributed throughout the body, we begin to look for intelligence, not just in the head and brain, but in our torso and extremities as well. Here it makes sense to talk about physical intelligence and what it means to have a "smart body." From a general point of view, we would say that a smart body is capable of a broad range of functional movement and knows how to avoid injury. More specifically, we can say that a smart body has good nervous system sensitivity and speed.

This physical intelligence begins with a form of sensitivity called proprioception. Proprioceptors are microscopic nerve cells located in skeletal muscles, joints, ligaments and connective tissue. These receptors monitor the degree of stretch and displacement in muscles and joints and notify the central nervous system of body positions and movements in space. This information is processed in the spinal cord and transformed into motor commands that tell the muscles when and how to contract. This feedback system is absolutely essential to physical function and performance.

The best way to understand how this system works is to picture your nervous system as a highly sophisticated, super-fast telephone network. Here's how it works: Suppose you've just stepped onto some uneven ground and your foot turns in an unexpected direction. This mechanical pressure stimulates the proprioceptors in your ankles, knees and hips. These cells call up the spinal cord and report their position and motion. They might say, "Hey boss, this joint is slightly flexed and it's rotating clockwise at an alarming rate. You'd better do something fast."

This information moves up the legs at astonishing speed, arriving at the spinal cord in a fraction of a second. When the spinal cord gets the call, it picks up the phone and makes note of the information. It then holds a meeting with other sensory neurons and attempts to integrate this information into an effective plan of action. This, unlike large-scale human meetings, happens with blinding speed and is generally very decisive.

Once the spinal cord arrives at a decision, it attempts to apply necessary corrections to the body in motion. It calls up individual muscles and stimulates them to contract in the correct order with just the right intensity. It says, for example, "Hey, quadriceps, wake up. We need you to maintain your contraction just a little bit longer, OK?" or "Hey calf muscles, if you would turn off just little bit sooner on the next step, we'll all be happier." If all goes well, the muscles will contract or relax as directed and smooth, balanced movement will be maintained or restored. The process is continuous, operating whenever the body is standing, walking, running or dancing.

If this communication process works smoothly and efficiently, the end result is graceful movement and the quality we call balance. Balance is not a single quality. Rather, it's a combination of sensitivity, speed and strength. In fact, we can say that balance is a communication skill.

Of course, if you've been on the couch for a few years, the communication process will sound somewhat different. The proprioceptors are dozing in their lounge chairs and may not even notice that your ankle or knee is rotated to a dangerous degree. If they do happen to notice, they'll take their sweet time calling up the spinal cord. But the spinal cord might be on vacation as well and the phone will be off the hook. If the spinal cord does get the message, it will procrastinate on getting the message out to the motor nerves. And of course, the muscles might not be paying attention either. Taken together, this all adds up to an unresponsive, injury-prone system.

It is easy to see why proprioception is such an important part of physical intelligence. Without proprioception, you wouldn't be able to perform any complex movements because you wouldn't know where your limbs were in space. Without proprioception, walking would be an extremely challenging task because you'd have to predict in advance how much to contract your muscles in every single stride. Poor proprioception makes for awkward, poorly controlled movement and greater injury. Without good proprioception, we would move like robots.

Good proprioception not only makes our bodies faster, stronger, and more stable, it also keeps us prehabilitated. Think about your ankle for a moment. Perhaps you've sprained it in the past or maybe there's been times when you've had a close call. Perhaps you stepped off a curb awkwardly and felt a sharp twinge. The difference between a close call and an actual ligament-tearing sprain is largely dependent on how fast your proprioception system is. If your proprioceptors are educated and awake, they will tell your central nervous system where your foot is in relation to your lower leg and this feedback will help to stimulate the proper leg muscles that will keep it in line. By having a good nervous system sense of ankle position, you avoid or minimize the injury.

Great athletes obviously have good proprioception, but so do other physical artists. Musicians have extremely high levels of proprioception–just imagine the violinist maneuvering up and down the neck with no frets to guide her hands. She can even do it with her eyes closed, using only the proprioception in her fingers, wrist, elbow and shoulder to guide her. Other great proprioceptive artists include dancers, sculptors and painters.

Proprioception is just as much a sense as vision and hearing and just as vital. Without proprioception, our bodies would be "blind" to position and movement and we would have no idea which muscles to fire, in what order or at what intensity. Some neurological disorders are characterized by a failure of proprioception. For people afflicted with this pathology, even the simplest movements demand a major effort of attention and concentration. Each move must be planned in advance and monitored consciously and continuously for error. Fast movement is out of the question. Balance becomes tenuous and injury likely.

Other individuals give up their proprioception willingly, through neglect and disuse. Spend a few decades on the couch and you won't really know where your body is in space. Suddenly, the skateboard that was once your friend is now a treacherous foe and the slippery surface in the bathtub is an outright menace. Use your proprioception or lose it.

Like our other senses, proprioception is trainable. If we challenge it consistently, we will become more adept at sensing where our limbs are and how they are moving. This should be an essential part of all physical education -having a smart body means having good proprioception. By improving your proprioception, you prehabilitate your body and decrease your chances of injury. Since you know where your limbs are and how they are moving, you will move more gracefully and efficiently. Good proprioception also correlates with the ability to heal after an injury has occurred. In fact, absence of pain is not enough; we cannot say that an injury has fully healed until proprioception has been fully restored.

In an effort to study proprioception in the shoulder, one researcher built a machine to measure rotation of the upper arm. He blindfolded his patients and asked them to say "Stop" as soon as they felt their arm moving. As we would expect, healthy patients could quickly detect movement of the arm, usually within a few degrees. But those patients with injuries to the rotator cuff were far slower in detecting movement; in some cases, the arm would rotate much further before the movement was detected. This finding has huge implications for functional movement. If you are slow to detect movement, you'll also be slow in contracting the muscles that protect the joint from excess movement. The lack of proprioceptive speed or sensitivity makes further injury more likely.

Like every other system in the body, proprioception is a use-it-or-lose-it system. If you don't ask your limbs to give you feedback about their position in space, they aren't going to do it; they're going to go to sleep. In other words, if you sit on the couch for a few years, your proprioception will atrophy, just like muscle tissue. Your appearance might not be a whole lot different, but your functional competence and injury resistance will be drastically reduced.

But now suppose that you finally decide to get moving and get in shape. Suppose you go out to play some tennis. Unfortunately, your ankle doesn't really remember how to judge it's own location; the sensitivity within your joints is way down because of disuse. But now you're loading up your body with vigorous ballistic motion and sure enough, your ankle is slow to recognize dangerous positions. By the time it tells the right muscles to contract and protect it, it's too late and you collapse like a wet bag of cement on the court. Too bad you didn't do some balance work before you got back into action.

Of course now you're really in for it because you're going to be back on the couch for a few weeks and your proprioception is going to decrease even more. The swelling around your ankle will limit the movement and so there's little chance to exercise any proprioception at all until you get some movement back.

my knee hurts, I'll make it smarter

This, by the way, sheds new light on the common approach to rehabilitation used by the typical amateur: "My knee hurts, it must be weak, I'll make it stronger by lifting weights." True, it might in fact be weak, and resistance work might help. But the pain might also be the result of poor coordination of nervous system elements. In this case, the more sophisticated approach is to emphasize the speed of communication between the afflicted body part and the spinal cord. Now you might say, "My knee hurts, it must be slow, I'll make it faster by working on my balance." This is not a total solution or a cure-all, but it is a step in the right direction.

the complete training program

To be considered truly holistic, a physical training program must include challenges to the proprioceptive system. In other words, we must put our bodies in positions that challenge us to listen to the positional feedback coming from our joints, ligaments and muscles. One of the best ways to do this is to intentionally put ourselves into precarious, unstable positions using toys such as physioballs, wobble boards and balance beams. This way, we'll be challenged to pay attention to where our body are in space.

In contrast, if you're strapped in to a rigid machine that is bolted to the floor, you take away the proprioceptive challenge and after awhile, that part of your nervous system goes to sleep. In this way, machines can actually de-train you and reduce your functional competence. Ask your personal trainer what she's doing to improve your proprioception; if he doesn't know what you're talking about, get another trainer.

In the meantime, take responsibility for your own training. Develop your proprioception by challenging your balance in diverse and unstable positions. Do all the balance work that you can. Use commercial wobble boards or make your own. When you go hiking, practice your balance by walking on fallen trees. At home, go to the park and find obstacles to stand on or jump over. Stand on one foot with your eyes closed. Or go out with a friend as a guide and do some walking with your eyes closed. Learn to control your body in space. A diversity of activity works well here because new activities always stimulate proprioception.

There are many ways to improve your balance. Start by playing kid's games, many of which are balance intensive. Imagine you're on a tightrope and walk a line on the floor. Go hiking and walk on irregular rocks and downed trees. Get a wobble board and invent some games. Or, stand on one foot and have your partner hold up her hands as targets. Your challenge is to touch her hands in alternation without falling over.

If you want to be disciplined and systematic about it, you can draw a compass rose on your floor, stand on one foot in the center and practice reaches to each of the main points, North, South, East and West. Or, you can try working with a partner/coach. The "athlete" stands on one foot while the "coach" applies light, harassing touches to the torso and hips. In this version, no hops are allowed. Simply keep the touches coming and disrupt the athlete's balance just enough to force them into an adjustment.

Wheelworks

These days, just about everyone knows that stretching and strengthening are important components of fitness. What is less widely known is how these two practices fit together in their combined effect on the body. In theory, we could educate ourselves by looking into the fine details of physiology and the microscopic effects of stretching and strengthening on muscle tissue. But if we try to approach this challenge by making a detailed analysis of all the factors and variables involved, we quickly get swamped in complexity and lose sight of the bigger picture. What we need is some kind of model to guide our understanding.

The bicycle wheel is ideal for this purpose. If you think in terms of muscles, tendons, and ligaments of the body, you'll see that the similarities are striking. Both the bicycle wheel and the musculoskeletal system are complex structures that depend on the combined length and strength of the individual elements. When the spokes are tensioned precisely, the load is shared across the entire structure and the wheel is "true." If any single part of the structure becomes short or weak, the entire structure becomes distorted and vulnerable to collapse.

Like the bicycle wheel, the human body has its share of problems and misalignment. That is, we sometimes have loose, sloppy or flaccid muscles and connective tissue; these are the loose spokes that fail to support the skeletal "rim" in motion. Other times we have rigid, short or tight muscles and ligaments; these tight spokes tend to pull the skeletal "rim" out of true. Stretching is the equivalent of loosening the spokes, strength training is equivalent to tightening the spokes. If you have loose or tight "spokes" in your body, you'll develop a "wobble," a distortion of your ideal movement pattern. In many cases, that wobble leads to pain, pain that can be difficult to diagnose and treat.

Of course, there are some pretty substantial differences between the bicycle wheel and the human musculoskeletal system. In the first place, the bicycle wheel is a two-dimensional structure that rotates on a single axis. When it goes out of balance, the rim can wobble either side to side (laterally) or in its distance from the center (radially) and that's about it. The human body, on the other hand is not only three dimensional, it is composed of many three dimensional, wheel-like sub-assemblies connected to one another. Thus, it is immensely more complicated than any bicycle wheel. This means that the number of possible wobbles–muscular imbalances that lead to pain–is basically unlimited.

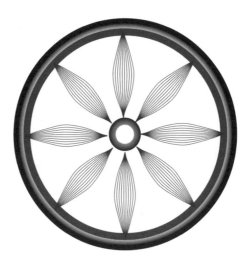

Not only that, spokes are inert and passive, whereas human muscles are capable of an astonishing range of finely-graded contractions. Our muscular spokes are controlled by a nervous system that is highly adjustable and subject to its own set of problems. So, there are some big differences between our model and the real thing, but for the sake of simplicity, let's ignore them for the time being.

Ideally, the human animal is born into the world with a neuro-muscular wheel that is "true" or nearly so. The body's musculature is not yet developed, but the potential for ideal length and strength relationships are in place. Give a child some diverse movement experience early in life and chances are his spokes will develop the ideal combination of length and strength that will keep his wheel rolling true.

This condition may hold for some years, even decades, but the combined effects of gravity, repetitious movement, injury and other influences will eventually cause a muscular spoke to tighten or weaken. A muscle may weaken because of disuse or injury; alternately, it may tighten because of disuse or to in an effort to protect an injured joint. In either case, one day you wake up and notice that your "wheel" has developed a "wobble." You may not notice the wobble itself–the misaligned movement pattern of your body can be extremely subtle–but you sure notice the pain that comes with it. Something is getting pinched, torqued, rubbed or pulled. You try ice and anti-inflammatory medications, but you still feel pain. So, you resolve to set things right again by truing the wheel. Maybe the right stretch or strengthening movement will get you back into alignment.

Unfortunately, the fitness world is sharply divided over how to treat our wobbly wheels. On one hand, the stretching advocate sees stretching as the universal cure for wobbles. He begins with the assumption that your wheel has tight spokes and prescribes a regimen of postures and movements to stretch them. Implicit in this assumption is the belief that muscles inevitably tend to become tighter over time and that stretching will ensure realignment. If you fail to get results, you need to stretch more. This method actually works on occasion because many people do in fact have lots of tight spokes. Unfortunately, there are many cases when it doesn't work at all; if the offending muscle is actually weak or loose, stretching might just make the wobble worse.

At the other end of the continuum, the strength training advocate sees resistance exercise as the universal cure for wobbles. He assumes that the wobble is due to flaccid, weak muscles and that strength training is the universal cure-all. He will instruct you in resistance exercises for all your spokes. If you fail to get results, you need to lift more weight or lift more often. This approach also gets occasional results because yes, many people do have weak, flaccid spokes that need to be toned and tightened.

What both of these approaches fail to realize is that any given body can have a combination of short and weak spokes and that methods that work for one condition won't work for the other. What we really need is an integrated, comprehensive approach to physical wheel-truing. If we could figure out precisely which tissues were tight and which were weak, we could create an ideal, customized program. Just stretch the tight ones and strengthen the weak ones and we'd be back in balance. Unfortunately, the problem with this highly targeted, muscle-specific approach is that, while it promises genuine effectiveness, it is also difficult and time consuming. It takes tremendous diagnostic skill to determine exactly which tissues are tight and which are weak.

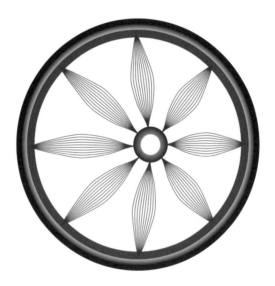

If you've ever tried to true a bicycle wheel, you know that it can be an exasperating, frustrating task; this is an art that can take years to master. But if truing a bicycle wheel is difficult, truing the human musculoskeletal system can only be described as hyper-difficult. There are hundreds of orthopedic tests for strength and range of motion. Hands-on evaluation of tight, loose and weak tissue requires decades to master. And, to make it even more challenging, these tests do not always yield consistent results between examiners. In other words, you can have 10 different physicians test a patient for, say, hamstring flexibility, and get significantly different opinions.

The other problem here is that weakness and shortness may be related in paradoxical, complex ways. For example, a muscular spoke might be both short *and* weak. If we simply stretch it, we might not make much progress. If we strengthen it however, it may gain improved function in a lengthened position which may allow it to readjust to its ideal length. In fact, many of today's coaches and therapists are coming to the conclusion that strength training is a vital part of increasing and maintaining flexibility.

The other problem in trying to repair the musculoskeletal problems of the human body is that the "spokes" do not respond anywhere near as quickly as we would like. With a bicycle wheel, the mechanic gets instant results. Just turn the wrench and the spoke gets tighter or looser, instantly. Spin the wheel and you'll see whether the wobble gets better or worse. So, it's relatively easy to discover the relationship between cause and effect, and with some trial and error we can learn to correct our mistakes. The feedback is fast and reliable.

In contrast, human "spokes" may not respond to truing exercises such as stretching and strengthening for weeks, months, or even years. Some nervous system adaptations are fast, but even for a young person in good condition, the effects of stretching and strengthening may not become evident for a long time. This situation is equivalent to turning the spoke wrench a half a turn and then waiting 6 weeks to see how it affects the wobble. Obviously, this turns musculoskeletal adjustment into an extremely laborious process that will try anyone's patience. It also explains why clinical care for musculoskeletal injuries is often extremely frustrating.

characteristic patterns

Given these challenges to truing the human musculoskeletal wheel, we might be tempted to throw up our hands and abandon the effort entirely; maybe we're just going to have to stick with the Tylenol and hope for the best. The good news is that there appear to be certain characteristic patterns of aging that hold true across most human bodies. Because of variations in muscle fiber composition and nervous system wiring, individual muscles perform and age differently. Some tend to tighten with age, others tend to weaken. Thus, we see characteristic patterns of distortion in the human body/wheel.

The pioneer in this study has been the legendary physical therapist Vladimir Janda. Janda took biopsies of muscle tissue from many areas of the body and found a distinct pattern of fiber types within each muscle. Some muscles are composed of a higher percentage of "tonic," or "slow-twitch" fibers. These muscles include the hamstrings, the pectoralis major, the upper trapezius, the psoas (the deep hip flexors that run from the lumbar spine to the upper leg), the inner thigh muscles, the calf, the biceps and the flexors of the forearms. In general, these muscles tend to shorten with age.

He also found that some muscles are predominately "phasic" or "fast-twitch." These include the abdominals, the butt, the middle and lower trapezius, the triceps, the rhomboids (between your shoulder blades) and the extensors of the forearms. In general, these muscles tend to weaken with age.

Janda's findings are routinely confirmed by the daily experience of physical therapists, doctors, athletic trainers and massage therapists, people who work with large numbers of aging human bodies. The profile that Janda describes fits older people perfectly. Just take a look at the senior citizens you see each day. You're likely to see a stooped, bent over posture, the logical result of short chest muscles and a weak upper back. You'll see a short stride because of tight hamstrings and calf muscles. You'll notice that they are slightly bent at the waist because of short hip flexors and you might also notice that their arms are bent at the elbow because their biceps are short.

If you were to assess their functional performance, you'd find that they can't jump very high or climb stairs very well because their butts are weak. And, if you talk to them for awhile, you'll find out that they're having a lot of back pain, due in some measure to the fact that their weak abdominals no longer provide support for their spinal columns. Some of these changes are due to lifestyle and to the individual's movement history, but a lot of it is straight-ahead, predictable muscle physiology.

Implications for physical training

Knowing what we know about the fiber composition of muscles and the variation that exists throughout the body, it would make sense to stretch those muscles which tend to shorten (the hamstrings, the pecs, the biceps, the calf, the psoas and the forearm flexors), just as it would make sense to strengthen the muscles which tend to weaken (the butt and the abdominals, most notoriously).

Unfortunately, almost no one is doing this. Most of today's exercise programs are blanket, one-method-fits-all methods that make no allowances for differences in muscle physiology and aging patterns. But since muscles respond differently to training, we can't just apply a single treatment or training method to all of them and expect to get good results.

Both yoga and weight training make this mistake, although from different directions. Yoga advocates assume that stretching is universally therapeutic and attempt to apply it to all the muscles of the body. A yoga instructor is considered knowledgeable if he or she knows a stretch for every muscle. But if you stretch every muscle in the body, you'll be benefiting some and wasting your time on others. There's not much to be gained by stretching muscles that tend to weaken with age. You'll simply end up with long, weak muscles.

Weight training advocates make a similar conceptual mistake when they assume that resistance training is universally therapeutic. A visit to the typical gym bears this out. We now see a machine for almost every muscle, the assumption being that all muscles need to be isolated, worked and strengthened. But if you do resistance training for every muscle in your body, you'll be benefiting some and wasting your time on others. There's not much to be gained by strengthening muscles that are already in the process of getting shorter. You'll simply wind up with a bunch of short, strong muscles. This adds up to a distorted posture, not a happy body.

Knowing what we now know about the various fiber ratios in our muscles, the more sensible approach would be to develop a hybrid discipline that attempts to target individual muscles with exactly what they need–stretching for the tonic muscles such as hamstrings, pecs and psoas, and strengthening for the butt and abs. As our understanding of muscle physiology deepens, we should be able to create highly specific exercises that, in combination, will counteract some of the posture-distorting effects of aging.

the long and short of stretching

In an effort to keep our musculoskeletal wheels true, many of us turn to stretching. Standard-issue fitness advice tells us that we need to stretch before and even after every exercise session. This guideline is held by the fitness industry as a standard for responsible, correct exercise instruction. Woe to anyone who fails to stretch and woe to anyone who fails to teach stretching.

Given the enthusiasm with which we promote stretching, one might assume that we know a lot about the subject. In fact, stretching is an extremely difficult subject to study objectively and we really don't know much about it. There are a huge number of variables involved in even simple stretches. Exercisers can vary the duration of the stretch, the number of muscles involved, the amplitude or intensity of the stretch, the frequency, the before and after conditions and so on. There are many ways to stretch and individuals show a lot of variation in the way they respond to stretching. Plus, nutrition, stress and hormonal levels can have a big impact on the flexibility of muscle and connective tissue. Clearly, men and women respond differently to stretching, as do adults and children

We could do laboratory studies, of course. We could take muscle, tendon and ligament tissue from rats or primates, place it on some sort of stretching device and measure how it responds. This may give us some interesting ideas, but it doesn't tell us anything at all about how stretching will affect tissues in living bodies. Or, we could take an experiential approach, trying different approaches to stretching and finding out what works. This is certainly worth the effort, but it also requires considerable diligence, patience and record-keeping. With so many variables, we'd need to hold most of them constant while we did our testing, something that doesn't always work so well in actual life.

Of course, we can always turn to the animal world for suggestions about how we ought to be stretching. We have all watched cats and dogs stretch and it seems safe to assume that their instinctual patterns are correct for their bodies. Since we share a large percentage of genetically-coded muscular physiology with these creatures, it is probably safe to assume that their methods are correct for our bodies as well.

So what do we see in other mammals and primates? In most cases, we see simple, short duration (1-5 seconds) stretches, straight forward and back in the sagittal plane. Every dog and cat owner knows this by routine observation. The animal wakes up, stretches his chest, his back and his legs and declares himself ready to go. These animals do not do complex, rotational postures or long duration stretching.

Yes, we do see that dogs do the yoga poses known as "downward dog" and "upward dog." The difference is duration. Whereas a yoga stretch might last from 5 seconds to a full minute or more depending on the teacher and the style, a dog will relax after a short stretch. This implies that we would do well to adopt a similar approach, integrating frequent, short-duration stretches throughout the day.

Of course, things may be different in a clinical setting where our goal is rehabilitation. If your body has been injured or has been sedentary for a long period of time, you may very well benefit from more aggressive, long-duration stretches of the affected tissues. But this is a specialized application. For routine living, the standard animal practice is probably appropriate and adequate.

the stretch reflex

When people think about stretching and flexibility, they usually think about short muscles that somehow become tight. But there's a lot more to flexibility than muscle and connective tissue; flexibility is actually a neuromuscular phenomenon. In other words, it has a lot to do with how the nervous system is behaving while the body is in motion. If we are to have any chance of understanding flexibility, we need to understand a circuit called the stretch reflex.

The stretch reflex is a nervous system feedback loop that links muscles with the spinal cord and higher brain centers. Tiny sensors within muscles are sensitive to stretch. When a muscle is stretched, these sensors send impulses up to the spinal cord where they synapse with motor neurons that stimulate contraction in the muscle that is being stretched. Thus, the more you stretch the muscle, the more it tries to contract. This circuit is adjustable and trainable, but we can safely ignore that fact for the time being.

The stretch reflex has two functions. In the first place, it is a protective mechanism. Obviously, a limb that is stretched too far is at risk of injury; stretch too far and you'll tear muscle tissue,

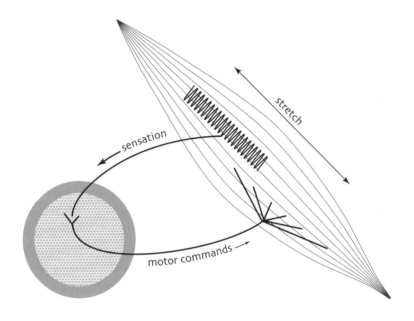

tendon and ligaments. The stretch reflex helps to prevent such over-stretched conditions. In this sense, this thing that we call the "stretch reflex" is actually an anti-stretch reflex. Without this kind of reflex, we would get injured on a daily basis.

Second, the stretch reflex helps us generate more powerful contractions in functional movement. Many movements that we do in our lives are composed of rhythmic alternations between stretch and contraction; the primal animal movement is an oscillation. Gait is a good example; muscles lengthen and then contract to propel us forward. When muscle lengthens to a certain point, the stretch reflex fires, which reverses the motion into contraction. If the stretch is vigorous, the stretch reflex can promote a powerfully elastic rebound movement. Thus, the stretch reflex is also a performance-enhancing mechanism. Without an active stretch reflex, we would have extremely poor athletic performance; we would be unable to move with speed or power.

In fact, this is precisely what is happening with so many physically uneducated people. Because they have little physical experience to draw upon, the stretch reflex doesn't fire at the right time. Either it kicks in too early, generating a low-amplitude, weak rebounding movement, or it kicks in too late, leaving the muscle and joint vulnerable to injury.

The key to improved physical performance and injury resistance is not simply increasing your range of motion. The key is figuring out how to get your stretch reflex synchronized with the movement in question. All physical arts, from music to dance to powerlifting, rely on accurate stretch reflex timing. In fact, we could go so far as to describe the entire athletic enterprise as an effort to tune stretch-reflex activity.

If we're trying to retain or improve our capacity for functional movement, we should try to preserve the protective and performance-enhancing qualities of the stretch reflex. Unfortunately, some stretch advocates consider the stretch reflex an adversary to be overcome in the quest for greater range of motion. In some clinical applications, we may need to push the stretch as far as possible, but in most cases, the stretch reflex is your friend. The goal in functional training is to get the stretch reflex perfectly coordinated with your actual muscle length and the activities you want to perform.

stretching and injury

Just about everyone in the fitness world now assumes that the practice of stretching will make us better athletes and help prevent injury. Given today's universal mania for this practice, we might assume that research has shown us clear, unequivocal results on the benefits of stretching for performance and injury resistance. In fact, they do no such thing.

The March 2000 issue of *Sports Medicine Digest* reviewed the research and found no support for the popular view. In particular, they reviewed a randomized trial performed on 1538 Australian military recruits. In this study, one group performed a standard series of warmup exercises alternating with stretches for major muscle groups. Subjects in the control group performed only the warmup routine which included jogging, side-stepping and other locomotor exercises.

After 12 weeks of rigorous training, the researchers found no statistically significant differences in the rate of injury between the two groups. The authors reported:

> There was no significant effect of pre-exercise stretching on soft-tissue injury risk or bone injury risk. A typical muscle stretching protocol performed during pre-exercise warmups does not produce clinically meaningful reductions in the risk of exercise-related injury.

From a biological standpoint, these findings make perfect sense. After all, we don't see non-human animals in the wild doing long-duration stretching routines. If cold-start movement really produced injury, animals who failed to warm up would have been eliminated from biological contention a long time ago. Wild animals often need to move spontaneously with speed and power; rarely do they have time to stretch before chasing prey or running away from threats. Animals that needed a stretching routine prior to moving would quickly be eliminated from the gene pool, having been eaten by those animals that don't need to stretch.

effect on athletic performance

Even as trainers zealously advocate stretching, researchers are discovering a profound lack of evidence to support it's supposed benefits. The *Journal of Strength and Conditioning Research* has published several articles in the last few years that are highly skeptical of stretching, especially as a warm-up. For example, the August 2001 issue carried a report, "Effect of Warm-Up and Flexibility Treatments on Vertical Jump Performance." The authors write "Despite the prevalence of athletes who engage in stretching routines before performing, there is a paucity of evidence that this actually enhances athletic performance."

In fact, there is clear evidence that under some conditions, stretching actually inhibits force production. In this particular study, the authors found a significant decrease in vertical jump after stretching. This makes sense; if we sedate the stretch reflex with long-duration stretches, we also lose some of its performance-enhancing qualities. We may get more range of motion, but that motion will be less coordinated, less intelligent and less powerful.

conclusion: focus on function

Given the number of mysteries surrounding stretching, it makes sense to stick with a functional orientation. Here we simply shape our stretching styles to match the physical objectives we are trying to achieve. In this case, our goal is to gain enough flexibility to meet the demands of our activities, sports or occupations. The goal is not flexibility for its own sake. Rather, stretching is a means to a functional end.

In normal human movements such as walking, running or climbing, we are continuously moving into and out of stretched positions. In the vast majority of cases, none of these stretched states last for more than a second, and in many cases, considerably less. If you consider the vast range of movements that humans typically perform, it is hard to think of any that require long-duration, stretched-out positions.

Ideally, our stretching ought to mimic the activities that we actually want to do. The idea is to duplicate, as closely as possible, the actual conditions where we need to develop greater range and ease of motion. So, instead of isolating a body part in some specialized, artificial manner, try to integrate a stretch into a normal, bipedal activity.

For example, you can perform an effective stretch while walking, simply by intentionally increasing the length of your stride. This promises better results than any abstracted or isolated stretching movement; after all, you're practicing a movement in which the timing, duration and depth of the stretch are perfectly matched to the objective.

Stretching is bound to remain a murky and confusing study without much in the way of hard facts or right answers. Nevertheless, there seems to be one thing that we can depend on–the importance of specificity. Instead of relying on some blanket prescription or formula, a better approach is to think about the functional demands that you are trying to prepare yourself for. It is not the case that you need maximum range of motion in all of your joints at all times. Surely the flexibility needs of the marathon runner are different from the flexibility needs of the gymnast. Thus it makes sense to target our stretching with as much precision as possible.

How you stretch depends on how you answer this question: does your activity demand mobility or stability in the joints in question? Will you need to move some part of your body to the limits of it's range, or will you want that area to be solid, stable and ready to withstand forces that might traumatize joints, ligaments and tendons? How you answer this question will determine the nature and timing of your stretching.

For example, let's say that you are going to go rock climbing. Climbing demands flexibility in the hips because it is often necessary to step high or wide. At the same time, the climber needs a high level of stability and dislocation-resistance in the shoulders. Consequently, it makes sense to stretch all the muscles around the hips, but go easy on the shoulders. In running, you would like to have good mobility in the hips to ensure a long stride, but excess mobility in the ankle could lead to ankle sprains. If you need stability, pump against some resistance to stimulate the stretch reflex and muscle activity around the joint. If you need mobility, go ahead and stretch.

Your approach should also take into consideration the nature of the joints themselves. The hip joint, being a deep ball and socket, is highly stable and dislocations are relatively rare. The shoulder, on the other hand, is a shallow joint, highly mobile and extremely prone to dislocation. On this basis alone, it makes sense to stretch the muscles around the hip joint, but leave the shoulder joint alone.

Pumping the compass rose

When physical therapists study therapeutic exercise, they are constantly on the alert for better ways to diagnose their patient's musculoskeletal disorders. Traditionally, the basic method has involved manual orthopedic testing. If a patient complains of pain in their knee, for example, the therapist can lay the patient down on a table, flex the patient's knee in several directions and try to determine precisely which tissues might be injured. This isolated manual testing method has become very sophisticated and can sometimes reveal the precise location of the problem, but as we are beginning to see, there are some serious limitations to this approach.

Even if we discover that a particular tendon or ligament is damaged or inflamed, we still might not know why. Sometimes the injury is the result of an obvious traumatic event, but it's also possible that the injury came on gradually, perhaps as a consequence of weakness or slowness in some other part of the body. It's not hard to imagine that a weak hip or dumb ankle could lead to a painful knee, for example. Even if we treat the painful tissue with ice and rest, the pain will probably return if we fail to address the true source of the problem. Thus, many physical therapists now try to look at the totality of the body in action.

In recent years, many physical therapists have begun using a simple floor pattern to test their patient's functional capability. The pattern resembles a compass rose, a circle with a center, some radial lines and cardinal points marked on the perimeter. Typically, the therapist asks the patient to stand in the center of the rose on one foot and perform a series of reaches, steps and hops. This allows the therapist to evaluate the patient's balance and body control in every direction.

These whole-body tests are proving to be extremely useful in diagnosing functional deficiencies. If a patient consistently shows poor balance in one direction or one plane of movement, we can assume that there's a muscular or neurological weakness. This naturally implies a strategy for correction. If your balance is really poor in a particular plane or direction, train yourself in that direction. If you're struggling with some sort of lower-extremity injury, you might reduce your pain by improving your functional performance where it is weakest.

This method of functional testing is extremely promising and is bound to become widespread in coming years. The problem however, is that physical therapists have applied a highly-specialized vocabulary to the process, thus limiting it's general adoption by average exercisers. In writing reports, for example, they might note that a patient demonstrated "poor posterior-medial balance." This is something an orthopedic physician can understand, but it also eliminates that chance that individuals might use this method for self-education or play. No one on the playground is going to challenge you to show off your posterior-medial balance skills.

It's much easier to simply think of the pattern as a compass rose or clock face and go from there. Stand in the center and test your balance. Reach to the east, then to the west. Note the difference. Touch the floor to the northwest, then reach high to the southeast. See how much you wobble. If you take a systematic approach, you may just discover a direction or a plane where you're weak. If you practice in that weak area, you will improve your overall balance and you just might find a solution to that nagging injury pattern you've been fighting.

Vigorous reaches and stepping moves on the compass rose will challenge most people, but if they prove too easy for you, you can increase the challenge by doing faster movements or by standing on a wobble board. Fast wobble board reaches will challenge even the most elite, world-class athlete. This arrangement also makes it possible for novices and experienced athletes to train right alongside one another in a class setting. The novice may struggle with a low-high reach from NW to SE for example, but if we add speed or a wobble board, the advanced athlete will struggle as well.

As you experiment with the compass rose, you'll also discover additional variations and games you can play. Try your reaches with a medicine ball, for example. If you factor in the various combinations of low, high, north, south, east and west, you'll find hundreds of possible movements. A really fun approach is to ask your training partner to hold up his hands as targets for your reaches; one hand high to the northeast, the other hand lower to the northwest, for example. Add in some variations and some heckling and you've got a good game going.

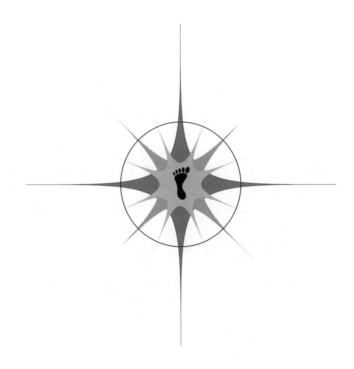

Don't get hurt in the first place

If you've ever been injured, you know the mantra "I never realized how much you use your hip (knee, ankle, back, shoulder) until I injured it. I can't do the things I like to do. All in all, I'd have to say that being injured just sucks."

Given the universally-agreed upon wretchedness of injury, one would think that we would have developed a strong understanding of injury-resistance and that we would spend a substantial amount of time actually practicing it. In fact, we have done nothing of the sort.

Part of the problem is cultural. When reflecting on the nature of health care, most of us reserve our greatest praise for heroic physicians who pull off spectacular, "miracle" cures. We worship those who conquer dread diseases and patch up broken bodies. In contrast, we have scarcely a word to say about people who prevent diseases and injuries. We don't give awards for injury prevention because success in this field is largely invisible; it is defined by things that don't happen.

This is a major oversight because prevention, although lacking in glamour, is really where the action is. Healing is a wonderful thing, but if we can avoid getting hurt or sick in the first place, we are far better off. Even if you're really adept at healing injuries and you've got the best medical care at your disposal, injuries extract a substantial toll. They interfere with our work and our play, they force our bodies to compensate in awkward patterns, and even worse, they make further injury more likely. Until you've really been injured, you won't have an appreciation for just how much it can disrupt your life. The pain is bad enough, but the loss of function is even worse. So, the obvious question is "What skills and qualities contribute to injury avoidance, prevention and resistance?"

injury resistance: general

General injury-resistance naturally depends on our overall state of fitness. Tissues that are adapted to frequent movement of any sort will be able to tolerate more stress. Muscles that are more endurant will be able to support more repetitions than those that fatigue after a few cycles. A nervous system that is experienced in making quick movement transitions will be able to hop, lean, shuffle or side-step percussive blows. In this sense, just about any conditioning program will increase your injury resistance. If you have a history of movement behind you, your body will simply be able to tolerate a wider diversity of abuse.

Some trainers suggest that we can increase our injury-resistance by increasing our "work capacity." This term refer to the volume of exercise that an individual can do over the course of hours or days. Modern coaches and therapists recognize that a high work capacity correlates with injury-resistance as well as the ability to heal quickly and effectively.

Please note that the term "work capacity" has nothing to do with the ability to push yourself through week-in, week-out 14-hour days at the office. What we're talking about is your ability to engage in sustained physical exertion, not your ability to produce reports, manage inventory or write software.

Notice also that the term "work capacity" makes no distinction between aerobic or anaerobic activity, or between strength and endurance activities. From this point of view, it doesn't matter whether you can run dozens of miles or do dozens of high-intensity squats in the gym; both require a large work capacity. The highly trained powerlifter, basketball player, rockclimber and triathlete all have a high work capacity, even though they use different physiological energy systems.

The significance here is that there appears to be a strong correlation between work capacity and the general ability of the body to resist injury and heal itself. Numerous stories of post-injury recovery by professional athletes suggest that a history of high-volume physical work simultaneously builds healing capacity. Top athletes heal well because they practice it; high volume workouts require frequent, microscopic healing. These athletes are good at self-healing because they challenge their bodies to do it frequently.

There are some distinctive patterns we see in work capacity over the course of an athlete's lifetime or career. Children, even the athletically gifted, have little work capacity. They can't maintain a high level of intense movement over a long session; they just don't have the physiological infrastructure in place to sustain it. Blood vessels don't deliver the necessary high volumes, mitochondria don't supply as much energy and the liver doesn't recycle metabolic waste efficiently.

It usually takes several years or as much as a decade to develop a high work capacity. Experienced exercisers and athletes who have already established a good work capacity don't need high-volume training; they can do better by emphasizing quality over quantity. Once you reach a point—for many athletes this occurs during their 30's and 40's—where work capacity peaks, it is best to concentrate on skill. If you've been working out all your life, you can safely assume that your work capacity is probably pretty good. You will still need occasional high-volume days to maintain that level, but since you've laid the foundation, you can proceed to high-quality play sessions that emphasize skill and quality. This is your reward.

But if you've been on the couch for a decade or so, you can safely assume that your work capacity is low and you're going to have to start building up some volume. At this stage, you'll be looking for a gradual, progressive increase in miles, yards, reps or sets. If your physical work capacity is low, you've got to put in the hours; there is really no other choice. Naturally, this is a delicate balance because increasing volume also puts you at increased risk of injury, but unfortunately, that's just the way it is.

specific elements of injury resistance

When we turn to specifics, we find that injury-resistance consists of several key elements. Obviously, simple strength will be a factor; strong muscles, tendons and bones are going to be more injury-resistant than weak ones. This is simple physics. Robust tissue can maintain its integrity even when challenged with above-average loads. It can withstand pulls, twists, shears, abrasions and impacts.

The good news is that we know how to make tissue stronger; load it up with cycles of significant resistance and repeat a few times a week. If you can make your strength training specific to anticipated injurious forces, so much the better.

Of course, traumatic events may not come all at once. Sometimes you'll fall out of a tree, but other injuries are the results of cumulative microtrauma that comes with hundreds, thousands or millions of repetitions that weaken tissue microscopically until it eventually fails. In these cases, injury resistance depends on a particular kind of endurance, the ability to withstand high numbers of movement cycles over the long haul. Obviously, you'll want to mimic the anticipated challenge by practicing similar numbers of repetitions.

Some people suggest that flexibility is a key factor in injury resistance, but others claim that excess flexibility is the bigger culprit. Actually, it's easy to imagine both extremes. If one part of the body's kinetic chain doesn't move all the way through its ideal range, and the athlete persists in an effort to execute the movement, the movement is going to have to come from somewhere. A movement restriction in one place shifts the stress onto another part of the body which may not be well-suited to carrying the load.

The fishing rod tells the story here: if one segment of the shaft is overly stiff, the movement will be concentrated in a smaller area, increasing the chances for material failure. Similarly, if the movement of your body is restricted by a tight muscle or joint, increased stress will be concentrated above and below the area of tightness.

On the other hand, we can see that excess flexibility in the kinetic chain can promote injury. This is especially true when there is inadequate speed, strength or endurance to control the movement around a joint. Motion without control is a recipe for musculoskeletal disaster. If one segment of the fishing rod is excessively soft, the motion will naturally tend to concentrate in that segment, which will inflict more stress on that material/tissue. Flexibility may be advantageous, but only if it is distributed evenly across the entire kinetic chain. The lesson? Don't concentrate your stretching on a single joint; distribute it widely.

Speed is surely the most neglected aspect of injury resistance; with the exception of some field sports, very few programs stress speed as important element in prehabilitation. Here I am not talking about macro, full-body speed, such as the ability to run 100 meters in 10 seconds. Rather, I am talking about micro speed, the responsiveness of individual parts of the neuromuscular system. I am talking about sensitive mechanoreceptors in joints, tendons and ligaments that send their messages up fast sensory fibers to a central nervous system that processes the message and sends it down a fast motor fiber to a wide-awake muscle fiber. I am talking about the ability to step off the curb, sense that your ankle is twisted slightly and apply a muscular correction before the load tears your ligaments.

Strong muscles may prevent injuries in some cases, but only if they contract fast enough to actually protect the joints that are being traumatized. Strong and slow doesn't really help us much. In fact, "weak and fast" may be a superior in terms of injury resistance, especially in highly dynamic situations.

It is surely the case that developing physical grace is strongly prehabilitative. Smooth movement in awkward conditions is something that we can practice and develop. And, if you're used to looking for grace in your movements, you'll be more likely to move smoothly when the injurious force strikes. The case in point here is dancer Gene Kelly. As an elite professional dancer, Kelly practiced smooth and graceful movement on a daily basis. And yet, over the course of a long career, he suffered almost no injuries whatsoever. Maybe he was just lucky, but I prefer to think that his well-practiced grace had a lot to do with it.

the paradox of prehabilitation

The paradox of prehabilitation is that, in order to effectively strengthen our bodies and make them more resistant to injury, we must actually expose ourselves to the forces that we are trying to build resistance to. This means that our training needs to be specific. That is, we must actually experience the things that will be injury-producing or biomechanically dangerous; otherwise, our physiology will not be stimulated to generate the precise tissue changes that we're looking for.

If, for example, you want to prehabilitate your knees against twisting, wrenching forces that tend to tear cruciate ligaments, you'll need to expose them to some degree of twisting, wrenching forces. If you want to prehabilitate your rotator cuff to high-speed acceleration and decelerations, you'll need to expose yourself to some degree of high-speed acceleration and deceleration. Given what we know about the specific adaptations created by the body, we can see that really is no other choice.

This approach sounds dangerous and in fact, it is. Excessive zeal in prehabilitation can cause injury. The key, of course is to expose ourselves to the anticipated trauma by degrees, to do it carefully and progressively. This requires a certain level of discipline and intentionality; this is where a good coach or physical therapist will be valuable.

All of our prehabilitative exercises can produce injury. In fact, they should produce injury, in very small amounts. That is the whole point of the enterprise. What we're trying to do is injure ourselves in tiny, microscopic increments so that in the long run we'll be able to endure truly challenging forces. The trick is to do it a little at a time.

personal

While general injury resistance is a good place to begin, we also need to narrow it down a bit and concentrate on the specific challenges that we face as individuals. Here you will need to make a study of the stresses that come with your particular lifestyle. What kind of movement demands come with your occupation or sport?

In addition, you must also consider your long-range functional objectives: what kind of activity do you want to engage in when you're 50? 60? 70? Do you want to be working in the garden? Then you must train for the squatting, lifting, cutting and carrying stresses that will you will place on your body. Do you want to be hiking in the mountains? With a pack? Over rough terrain? Then this will set your training and prehabilitation schedule.

Once you have studied the physical challenges that you will most likely be encountering, build in a margin of error to protect against the unknown. Add breadth and depth to the formula: diversify around whatever quality you are training for. If your functional objective requires say, endurance, train for a little more endurance than you really need. The same holds for other qualities such as balance, agility, strength or sensitivity. Concentrate your efforts on the most likely challenges, but don't specialize too narrowly. Diversity itself has a prehabilitative effect because it forces the nervous system to use different patterns.

In any case, all of this will involve a certain amount of effort. If you want to play hard, you've got to push the tissue. Otherwise, it's just going to go dormant. Still, even at this, the effort is still worth it because, it's a lot more pleasant working hard in an uninjured state than it is trying to work injured tissue back into shape. The choice is simple: you can sweat a little now or you can suffer a lot later.

Playful:
jumping for joy

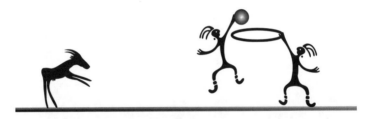

The power of play

Most people have overestimated how much money they need and have miscalculated the work-to-play ratio...Except us.

Tom and Ray Magliozzi
Car Talk

In our quest for improved physical fitness, many of us have been asking the wrong questions about our bodies. People with a cosmetic orientation ask "How good can I look?" Those with an athletic orientation ask "How can I beat the competition?" People with a medical orientation ask "How can I stave off dread diseases?"

These are not bad questions, but in terms of promoting widespread improvements in human health, they are not really on target. The questions we ought to be asking are "How gracefully can I move?" "How vigorous can I be?" "How good can I feel?" and perhaps most importantly, "How much fun can I have in the process?"

Play is the most underrated part of the modern physical education experience. Play is for kids, so we're told. Work is for adults. Woe to any adult who actually admits to playing. Play is considered frivolous, unproductive, selfish and self-indulgent. It has no validity and no justification. This bias against play is so pervasive that the only way we can get away with play in today's world is to disguise it under a cloak of labor or sporting achievement. If you want to move your body in public, be sure to call what you're doing a "work-out," lest anyone question your motives.

Opponents of play are suffering from an excess of gravity. Nose to the grindstone and fingers to the bone. Stop playing and grow up. Results are what matter. Just get it done. Achievement is paramount. The grim warrior wins the battle. I labor, therefore I am.

In today's fitness world, this pro-work, anti-play orientation approaches a clinically significant psychosocial disorder. Play is essential to animal wholeness and must be considered part of a complete education at all levels. Living without play is not a noble and commendable approach to life, it is a deficiency and an aberration. Absence of play is not a sign of maturity, it is a sign of pathology.

Anti-play zealots tell us that achievement and tangible results ought to be our primary concern. They instruct us to get back to work and get the job done. But even here, they miss the point. That is, play is not only intrinsically valuable for a complete and fulfilling life, it also helps us get the job done. When conducted with a little imagination and intelligence, play has profoundly beneficial effects on the human nervous system and in turn, on all levels of performance. Play not only makes us happier people, it also makes us more productive workers. In other words, play is not only fun, it's functional too.

Many Americans find this idea of legitimizing play difficult or impossible to comprehend. We are obsessed with work; we reflexively assume that the best way to get in shape is to do something called a "work-out." Presumably, this term is a consequence of our Puritanical roots and a by-product of industrialization. Naturally, it implies the need for labor, as in those cases when a relationship goes bad and we have to "work it out." According to this orientation, if you've got a problem, labor is the solution.

As it so often happens, language determines our attitude as well as the result. If you call it a "work-out," you're going to enter the experience with a set of assumptions, namely, that movement is labor. This work ethic leads directly to a "work-out ethic," a belief that the amount of work performed is the measure of the person and that more is necessarily better. Obviously, this is not a good place to begin a physical training program. If we start physical education with the word "work," it's not hard to understand that people fail to get excited.

the benefits of physical play

The benefits of play are both broad and deep; broad in the sense that a playful attitude can give us pleasure across a wide range of

activities and interests, deep in the sense that play can be truly profound.

On a physical level, all of the well-established benefits of exercise also come to us with physical play. We've all heard the list by
now: increased cardiopulmonary function, improved strength and
endurance, greater flexibility, coordination and balance. Whatever
exercise gives us, play can also give us.

Yes, in a strictly scientific sense, play might not always deliver the
ideal kind of movement for elite athletic fitness. If you're scamper-
ing around the field, starting and stopping erratically, you might not
keep your heart rate in the target zone continuously and you might
not do enough sets and reps to stimulate major tissue changes.

But in the real world, play trumps the scientifically correct methods for the simple fact that people are more likely to actually do it.
Play can give us many of the benefits of laborious exercise, but it can
also give us something that most workouts cannot; a sense of joy
and elation. And in non-human animals, play delivers just fine. The
playful dog doesn't do sets, reps or check his heart rate, for example;
he gets in shape entirely without labor.

The other wonderful thing about play is that it levels out our
social hierarchies as it makes physical education more egalitarian.
Success in play is a personal judgment call; no one can rank our
performance, no one can claim alpha status as the "most playful"
and no one can put us down. There can be no MVP, no top 10, no
Hall of Fame. You get to make the call on the quality of your own
experience. If you're having fun, you're doing it right.

Being subjective, play can't be measured, broken down or analyzed. There can be no stats or spreadsheets. No Olympic finals in
play, no standings, no rankings. Fun is in the body and the spirit
of the player, not in the eyes of the judges or on the faces of stop-
watches. There can be no standards, no qualification rounds, no
eliminations; just experience. No shoe contracts to the best players,
no endorsement deals to those who get the most pleasure out of
movement. It's up to us; we get what we play for.

it's not just for kids

A common assumption among hard-core exercise fanatics is that while play is fun and possibly valuable, it just isn't physically demanding enough for adult conditioning. After all, if kids are the ones doing it, it must be easy, right? There's no sustained aerobic challenge here, no major resistance to movement and thus no authentic training effect. Play is just kid stuff.

From a conventional point of view, this might be true. If we looked at play from the perspective of exercise science, a typical session might not measure up to what we need for serious adult conditioning. Playful bouts of intermittent pursuit, evasion, mock combat and other child-like movements might not burn big calories or generate enough resistance to stimulate cardiovascular fitness. Consequently, we might be tempted to dismiss the whole thing outright.

The problem is not with play itself; the problem is that we haven't created play forms that meet our adult needs. We haven't increased the challenge. It's not that play is inadequate; rather it's that we haven't created the kind of play that we need.

With today's new exercise toys, creating such adult play is actually a simple matter. By using such devices as medicine balls, physio balls and hula hoops, we can create games that are not only playful, but that will challenge the most hard-core fitness buffs. All it takes is a little imagination. If tag is too easy, play it on a hill. If hop scotch doesn't challenge you adequately, spread out the course and add more obstacles. If a game of catch doesn't pump you sufficiently, use a medicine ball. And if that's still not enough, stand on a wobble board. Any children's game, if tweaked in a creative fashion, can be a positively anabolic, heart-pounding experience.

it's self-reinforcing

Because so many of our exercise programs are inherently monotonous, many exercisers and would-be exercisers go looking for motivation. After laboring for a few weeks or months, we find that we need some kind of extra stimulus to get us off the couch and down to the gym or out onto the track. We listen to motivational speakers, buy motivational books, listen to motivational music and drink motivational beverages. It's curious that we should need so much stimulation for something that is supposedly natural. We assume that the problem is our own lack of ambition, but the fact that we're looking for external motivation suggests that there's something wrong with the activity that we're trying to get motivated for. We need external motivation because the common exercise program consists of dull, laborious repetitions; in other words, work.

Imagine the difference if our exercise programs were more play-centric. Imagine the difference if the program itself gave us the motivation to show up and get moving. There would be no need for external motivation—no motivational speakers, books, tapes or beverages. The power of play lies in the fact that it gives us instant pleasurable feedback. We play because it feels good and because it feels good, we want to play more. We don't do it because we should do it; we do it because we want to do it. The activity itself contains its own reward. What an excellent arrangement!

Varieties of play

Play is devilishly difficult to define. If we take a broad view, we might say that, like art, play is "what we do when the chores are done." Or, we might even say that like art, play is "whatever you can get away with." These definitions are fun to consider, but they basically leave the question wide open. So let's narrow it down by creating some categories. Students of play are likely to identify three basic varieties; primal play, practical play and free play. In practice, these varieties of play overlap considerably and often coexist simultaneously.

primal play

Primal play is the kind of play that young animals do to prepare for their adult lives. Typically, we think about carnivore cubs that "play" at hunting by wrestling with one another. Or, we might think of young herbivores who chase and dodge, "playing" at escape and evasion. This kind of play is not consciously intentional, but it is highly functional. The animal that plays in youth is far better prepared to face the challenges of adulthood. For animals in the wild, this is literally a matter of life and death.

Primal play is invariably physical; there is no ambiguity here. We see all the qualities that we normally associate with modern physical fitness training: strength, agility, endurance, balance and flexibility. This form of play is highly vigorous and challenging. Since much of this movement involves direct contact with other living animals, participants are forced to higher levels of performance. There is pleasure here to be sure, but there is also a sense of urgency and intensity. This kind of play is fun, but it's no laughing matter.

There are several safe assumptions we can make about primal play. First, we can assume that the playful movement patterns favored by young animals are appropriate to their bodies and are consistent with their evolutionary origins. The natural world is ruthless in selecting out individuals with inappropriate physical behaviors. Any young animal that played at inefficient or inappropriate movements would be unlikely to make it to reproductive age.

We can also assume that the playful movement patterns favored by animals are likely to be biomechanically and neurologically correct for their bodies. The movements that feel good are probably ideal for long term, pain-free function. From an evolutionary point of view, it would be truly bizarre if it were any other way. Any animal that had to struggle against unpleasant sensation to learn basic movement skills would simply not get very far. We can also assume that these primal, inborn play patterns are likely to prehabilitate animals against future injury. Bouncy, playful physical movements strengthen muscle tissue, bones, tendons and ligaments. They also help the sensory and motor nervous system to synchronize with the natural elasticity of the body.

The primal play that humans engage in is similar to that of many other species. Typically, we do a lot of combative play when we're growing up, testing movements of attack and evasion, lunging and retreat. Children typically wrestle, tickle and spar with one another. The play impulse says "You chase me for awhile, then I'll chase you." We can assume that these movements are adaptive to life on the grassland and would prepare young hominids for contact with other creatures, both human and non-human.

As the young animal grows, primal play is gradually replaced by more goal-directed behaviors such as hunting, predator avoidance, grazing and mating. As animals mature, they are forced out of their parent's care and into the world at large. Play is gradually transformed into essential behaviors such as actual pursuit and evasion.

From this observation, we might assume that play is strictly for kids. But we also know that, if the animal is fortunate enough to live in a safe environment, play will continue throughout life. Dog owners know this from casual observation. A dog that's abused will stop playing at an early age. But if you provide safety and basic comfort, that animal will continue playing throughout his or her life. Barring injury or abuse, dogs will keep playing until their bodies break down.

practical play: play as a means to an end

Practical play is goal directed, a means towards an end. Here we find that play can be a highly intentional and effective means to a functional or aesthetic end. Play prepares the nervous system for sophisticated movements and can thus increase our skill in any activity. If practiced in the proper proportion, we can use play to increase our performance across a whole host of disciplines.

Suppose you get a new tool in your workshop or your art studio that you haven't used before. You've got a fair idea of what it can do, but before you can really exploit its capabilities, you've got to get some sense of what is possible. You don't want to just take it out of the box and use it straight away on an important project; you want to test its strengths, weaknesses and limitations.

You could read the manual, but that's not going to help much. A better way to gain familiarity is through play. Manipulate it, feel it's qualities, try a few impulsive strokes, make a mess. In the process, you'll build up a neurological sense of its size, weight and stability. After this playful trial period, you're in a much better position to use it skillfully.

In this way, we begin to see an obvious sequence for skill development; that is, play before work. This is particularly the case if we're trying to do delicate or high performance work. The more we can build our neurological familiarity through play, the better our work performance will ultimately be.

In this way, we can actually use play as part of intentional strategy to improve individual and organizational performance in just about any endeavor. Here we actually design in play periods. This is particularly valuable in today's culture where innovation is relentless. New products and methods are constantly coming into use, challenging our ability to learn and adapt. In this sense, play is more important now than it has ever been. Today's worker can't simply coast on the skills he developed during his apprenticeship; he has to learn new methods almost constantly. And thus, he's got to play.

In the worlds of art and music, we often hear teachers give instruction that is based intentionally on play. Typically, they explain the basic elements of a concept or a technique, then instruct their students to try it out. "OK, now mess around with it." In other words, now that you've received some training in the fundamental concept or movement, it's time to innovate, create options, try new combinations and explore the boundaries. There is a rhythmic pattern to this process: Instruction, then play. Direct attention, then play. New concept, then play.

free play: play as an end in itself

The third variety of play is free play. This is strictly for pleasure, an end in itself. This kind of free play is spontaneous and improvisational. We do it for one simple reason, because it feels good; it has no evolutionary justification. It is not scripted, regimented, or packaged. It's not done by rote or formula. Beyond simple pleasure, there is no objective. It's not done by the numbers or in any particular sequence. It has no affiliation with any particular school or style of practice. There can be no evaluation or performance standards. Success in this kind of free play is judged entirely by the individual who is doing the playing.

In free play, we find a place where we're safe and comfortable and allow our bodies the freedom to do exactly what they want. Free play is authentic movement, pure expression of who we are and what we're feeling. This free play may seem frivolous to some, but it is absolutely necessary to good health and quality of life.

Free physical play is not unlike the comedic improvisations we see on stage or the musical improv of jazz, blues and rock musicians. The idea is to take some sort of riff or theme and go with it. The challenge is obvious; you don't really know where you're going, but you keep moving anyway.

In physical play, we start with a basic movement and expand on the theme. A simple hop is pretty boring, but what if you add some lateral movement or some rotations? What about a helicopter hop or a slalom hop? What if you add some leaning and some twisting?

You might make a fool out of yourself, of course. The comedian might make a lame joke, the musician might come up with a riff that is dissonant or dull, and the movement combination you invent just might be awkward or weak. You could play it safe, of course, and just stick with standard-issue sets and reps. If you just do bench press, you'll be safe.

In playful movement, this means changing speeds, amplitudes, direction and emphasis. Naturally, there's going to be waste in the process. A lot of your movements will be awkward, jerky combinations that you won't want to repeat. But if you put yourself slightly off balance and go towards innovation, you increase the chances of creating something meaningful.

Making a mess is a time-honored, proven technique for solving problems and extending the field of knowledge. Of course, as with any creative process, you've still got to edit your performance. Inevitably, your mess-making effort will generate a few gems, a few possible keepers and a whole lot of noise, trash and debris. Therefore, you've got to make some choices, picking out the good ones and throwing everything else away.

There will also be risk. If you go really wild in making a movement mess, you might twist your ankle or throw out your back. Of course, you might also create a movement that brings you great joy and satisfaction.

how to

Given the nature of the subject, the idea of a how-to instruction manual for play seems ludicrous. Unfortunately, given the state of the modern human body, it also seems necessary; we need this remedial education.

The basic instructions are simple: First, take a simple movement that you find interesting or pleasurable; it might be something as innocent as a guitar chord or as outrageous as a 6 foot high jump. Do some repetitions to make sure that you've got the basic movement mastered. Repeat the movement with enough frequency so that you can perform it reliably and without significant error.

Now start playing. Take the basic movement and put some life into it; animate it. Mess with the timing; stretch it, then contract it. Put some bounce into it, then add some swing. Take it apart and scatter the pieces around, then put them back together in some fresh combination. Put your own interpretation into it. Personalize it; give it your unique expression.

Above all, make it three-dimensional. Find the places where it's linear and make it rotate. Find the places where it's stagnant and make it breathe. Get audacious. Don't just pluck the strings of the instrument or the muscles of your body—bend the notes. Find out how far you can distort the tone while still maintaining the essential character of the original movement. Make up variations and recombinations as you wish; do it backwards, sideways and upside down. Follow the juiciest variations where they lead. Dance the movement; if you don't know how to do what you're after, bluff. Pretend that you know where you're going. Keep branching out with variation until you exhaust your interest or find the notes that you've been looking for.

transcending scales and chords

In learning how to play, physically-minded people can take a lesson from the musicians. Regardless of style, most musicians follow a basic learning progression. First they learn the fundamental scales and chords on their instrument, then they start improvising and playing with the myriad combinations. Scales and chords can be interesting in and of themselves, but no one wants to linger too long on these fundamentals; there is too much fun to be had by moving to the next level.

For the physical educator, sets and reps are the scales and chords of the body's music. Grab a dumbbell and do some presses. A set of ten will give you the basic idea, but that's not a magic number. If your movement is wobbly and weak, the chord is dissonant; you need to practice more. If your movement is assertive and competent, it may be time to move on to something more, well, musical.

Yes, we can analyze the biochemistry of sets and reps. We can say that so many reps and so many sets will produce a certain kind of anabolic response in muscle tissue. We can say an individual needs to do a certain number of sets and reps for weight loss and another combination for building muscle mass and so on. But in a way, this misses the point, just as if we told a young guitar player that he had to do a thousand major scales a week because the laboratory studies said so. The pleasure that comes from skillful execution is the goal. Repetition is simply a means to that end.

Sets and reps are entry level. They prepare your muscle tissue and nervous system for play, in the same way that chords and scales prepare the musician for play. There is nothing wrong with specializing in scales and chord or sets and reps, but there is so much more out there to be enjoyed.

Play in three dimensions

If physical play is anything, it is three-dimensional. It swings, rotates, slides and dances. Never linear or robotic, it twists and reaches, turns and rolls. In the language of the physical therapist, we say that play is multi-joint and multi-plane.

When studying the movements of the human body, specialists often refer to the three primary planes: sagittal, frontal and transverse. In simple terms, this means that we can move front to back, left to right, or with twists and rotations. The football kicker swings his leg in the sagittal plane, we do jumping jacks in the frontal plane, and discus throwers and belly dancers do their movement in the transverse plane.

Movement specialists use this kind of nomenclature because it helps them to categorize various human movement types and allows them to identify patterns and relationships between structure and function. A certain muscle group, for example, might be most active in the frontal plane or a particular injury pattern might be more common in the transverse plane. By studying the body in this way, these professionals discover ways to improve athletic performance and rehabilitation.

In practice, it's actually rare to find a human movement that takes place exclusively in one plane. Most functional movements, especially those that relate to hunting, gathering and athletics are combinations of movement–in many cases, they are diagonal or spiraling movements that take place in several planes simultaneously. Even walking and running, although they appear to be strongly single-plane movements, actually involve extremely subtle combinations of tri-planar movement.

Unfortunately, many of today's conventional exercises and calisthenics are performed in one plane, most typically the sagittal plane. Similarly, most exercise and weight-lifting machines limit our movements to a single plane. Stationary bikes, lat pull down machines and knee extension machines are all single plane devices. Rarely do we see an exercise machine that works multiple planes.

Body building movements are also notoriously single-plane. Curls, quad extensions on the machine, bench press, triceps extensions, crunches and lat pull downs—there is no rotation in any of these movements and thus no athleticism and no sense of play.

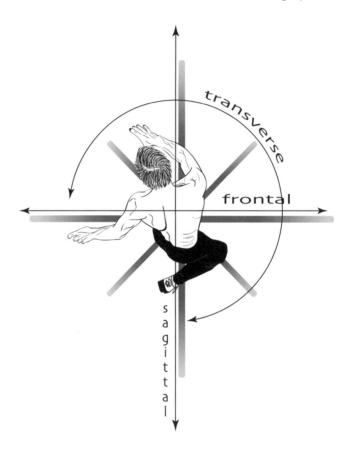

It is also worth noting that the single-plane movement style is extremely common in militarized cultures. Goose-stepping military marchers and drill teams move almost entirely in a single plane. The emphasis is on disciplined precision and synchronization. Marching troops, honor guards and the presentation of weapons are usually straight-ahead, direct and assertive. These are sagittal styles.

In contrast, dance is universally 3-dimensional and multi-plane. Belly dancing is strongly multi-plane, but so are modern, jazz and ballet styles. A good dancer is someone who can move through all planes simultaneously, without getting stuck in a single kinetic rut. He can take a single plane movement, add some rotation and take it into another plane without hesitation. In fact, we usually recognize a poor dancer as someone whose movements are limited to a single plane and who finds it difficult to transition to other planes. If you want to dance well, start exploring the frontal and transverse planes.

the athletic ideal

The athletic ideal of graceful human movement is 3 dimensional. What we're looking for in athletics is multi-plane competence. We see this in the gymnast's routine on the pommel horse, in the point-guard's shifting, supple drive to the basket and in the wide receiver's corkscrew leap for the touchdown pass. It is particularly evident in the martial artist's punch; a strong transverse movement of the torso drives the strike, just as a rotating crankshaft drives a piston. The punch looks sagittal, but is actually highly transverse.

From a functional standpoint, our objective is to develop strength, speed and endurance in all planes. This leads us to a working definition of athleticism: the ability to move through all 3 planes with power, grace and fluidity.

the transverse plane

For sport and living, the least emphasized but most important physical skill is competence in the transverse plane, the spiral and rotational movement. The transverse plane is unique because it is not under the direct influence of gravity. Gravity can pull you forward or back (sagittal plane) and it can pull you left or right (frontal plane), but unless you are in an unusual position, it will not pull you transversely.

Transverse plane movements are powered in large measure by the abdominals, especially the obliques. Working diagonally between your pelvis and rib cage, these muscles provide an essential functional connection between the lower and upper body. If that connection is tight, strong and fast, your overall movement is likely to be athletic. If the connection is loose, slow or weak, your movement is likely to be awkward, inefficient and injury-promoting.

play in all 3 planes

One way to make movement more playful is to take boring single-plane movements and make them more complex and multi-planar. Instead of just lifting the dumbbell straight up or straight out, see if you can find a way to put some rotation into the movement. Instead of doing a standard, straight-ahead squat, see if you can create a variation that turns or spirals. In particular, study the way that your abdominal obliques work as diagonal movers across your torso. By creating these variations, you'll not only make your training more functional and effective, but you'll have a lot more fun as well.

Sensation before numbers

Everyone has their own style of exercising, but these days, many people have come to assume that record keeping is essential to success. This is particularly obvious in the worlds of weight training, running and swimming, where participants go so far as to log every rep, every lap and every mile on custom-crafted spreadsheets, tabulated and cross-referenced down to the last variable. A good day is judged by good numbers, a bad day by poor numbers.

From our playful perspective, this approach doesn't make a whole lot of sense. True, numbers can be valuable. If you're trying to wring the greatest possible performance out of your body, you'll want to make your training as scientific as you possibly can. Obviously, accurate measurement is essential to this process. If you want to test your theories about what works, you've got to have some numbers to work with, some quantities that you can compare and observe for change. Maybe you have a theory that you'll swim faster when you kick with a certain cadence or that you'll develop more speed by doing interval work. Without numbers, this will all be guesswork; your program can drift aimlessly and you may not be sure how you're really doing.

Unfortunately, there are some serious problems with this data-intensive approach. In the first place, it completely violates our heritage of hunter-gatherer athletics. We can say with complete confidence that, prior to the invention of numbers, paper and clipboards, no hominid athlete ever kept track of miles, laps, sets or reps. But a lack of data did not compromise their performance in the slightest. Similarly, non-human animals don't keep track of anything either and they seem to do quite well. Clearly, numbers aren't necessary for performance training or health.

The other problem with health and fitness data tracking is that once we get started, it's impossible to know when to stop. As we

220

know, heath consists of many interdependent variables. Ideally, if we wanted to make the maximum possible progress in health and fitness, we would quantify every dimension of our lives and training. We'd measure and record everything, from calories consumed to miles walked to weight lifted. We'd keep an aerobics journal, a stretching record, a dietary log and a sleep record. And since stress is a major component of health and fitness, we'd log all the data about our relationships, including work, family and friends. Of course, if we did all these things, we wouldn't have time for much else.

The biggest problem with the clipboard-driven style is that it interferes with our sense of play. Record keeping is a bother and a distraction; it is labor. It takes us out of the movement and flow we are trying to enjoy. The mere act of logging numbers can transform even the most pleasant physical enterprise into labor. From this perspective, we can see that taking a clipboard to a movement session is almost as bad as taking a clipboard out on a romantic date. Sure, if you tracked all your numbers, you might increase your performance, but you'd really be missing the point.

We can see the same chilling effect that data-driven youth sports has on children's play. As soon as we start keeping score, logging stats and tracking victories, we violate the spirit of simple exuberant movement. We take children out of their bodies and turn them into physical accountants.

In most cases, personal record-keeping is not really compatible with sane and practical living anyway. Do you really have the time to write down every snack, every exercise and every vitamin supplement? Are you really going to put a stop watch to your stretches or measure every mile you walk? If you have a personal trainer on call, you might be able to manage such a program, but for most people, such detail is absurd. Our exercise and training sessions should give us relief from the labor that we are obliged to perform on the job each day; who wants to add another layer of work to an already over-worked life? At some point, fitness record keeping becomes a neurosis, not a health-promoting activity.

The rub here is that in terms of pure physical education, record keeping is a side show and a distraction anyway. Numbers are abstractions that exist only in the mind; the body knows nothing of numbers. There are no nervous system receptors in your body that track the number of reps, sets or miles. No such sensors exist because no such sensors are needed.

What the body does understand is sensation. We have a vast array of nervous system receptors that sense chemical concentrations, mechanical pressure, movement and pain, but not numbers. We can sense how much lactic acid is concentrated in our tissue, how much a muscle is stretched and whether a joint is slightly flexed or rotated. These are the things we can know, and if we are striving to become physically educated, this is where we ought to concentrate our attention.

This has always been the case throughout human evolution. Our hunting and gathering ancestors never counted sets or reps. They never measured distances. There were no laps. They probably had some sense of speed as in "it takes a day to go to the upper valley and back," but that was only a marker, not something to be striven for in and of itself. And yet, despite this complete lack of numerical accounting, these individuals managed to achieve a level of fitness far beyond what most of us achieve today. Obviously, numbers are not necessary for fitness.

Consider the difference in a modern context. One person goes running and sets a personal record for speed at his favorite distance; he feels a sense of achievement for having done so. Another person doesn't bother to bring a stopwatch, but pushes hard anyway and comes away with a fresh understanding of how his muscles feel when they're saturated with lactic acid. Which person is more physically educated?

If you're going to keep records, do it in the service of testing your ideas about what works. One of the craziest things you can do is to write down all your sets, reps and miles, just for the sake of writing them down. The act of writing down information, by itself, will never improve your performance or your enjoyment. In fact, given what we know about the SAID principle, we know that writing down numbers will only improve your ability in one task: writing down numbers.

Better yet, just forget about numbers. Counting takes you out of your body. Instead, concentrate on the quality of your movement and pay attention to how your body feels as you become fatigued. Start with smoothness and graceful execution. Your first few reps may be a little rusty, but you should get into the groove pretty quickly. Once you get the rhythm, keep emphasizing smooth movement. Once your smooth movement is well established, start adding power, speed and authority to the movement.

Of course, you can only maintain this for so long before fatigue sets in. When you feel the onset of fatigue, redouble your efforts for smooth and graceful movement. Your power and speed will naturally diminish as lactic acid builds, but don't sacrifice the quality of your movement.

In practice, concentrate on your playful spirit. Stop counting and start listening to your body; pay attention to sensation before numbers. Stop measuring and start observing. Stop calculating and start improvising.

Toys

We have no idea what the earliest toys were like. Surely they were organic in nature; wood, stone, bones or shells—these things tend not to fossilize. Neverthless, it's easy to imagine Paleolithic kids going wild with springy tree limbs, pestering one another and launching projectiles. In fact, it's not hard to imagine that the ubiquitous bow and arrow probably came directly from hominid play.

Tree branches may be fun, but they are a natural given. The first actual hand-made toy might have been a simple ball, maybe a bit of leather wrapped around itself, then stitched crudely together. This invention must have caused quite a stir on the Paleolithic playground; we can imagine kids and adults flocking from all across the savannah to see and play with the new thing. It must have been great fun; you could throw it like a rock, but it wasn't so hard. Plus, it felt good in the hand. Suddenly, all sorts of movement opportunities opened up. Throw, run, catch, kick. Academic researchers tell us that tools, fire and language were the key developments in the evolution of human intelligence and consciousness. But maybe it was just a ball.

what makes a good toy?

In the movie *Big*, Tom Hanks played a child who magically came to inhabit an adult body. Fortuitously, he is hired by a toy manufacturing company and becomes a consultant in toy design. In one memorable scene, Hanks meets with play-deprived company managers and explains to them how to design a good toy.

If Hanks' character was our consultant in designing exercise and fitness toys, I imagine that he would list a few key qualities: they should be simple and indestructible, they should bounce and roll and they should be adaptable to many possible uses. They should be designed in such a way that you'd want to touch them, throw them and jump on them.

Specifically, we're looking for toys that get us moving, toys that stimulate us towards vigorous, whole body play. They should be versatile so that we can invent new games with them. They should challenge our stability, our core body strength, our agility and our locomotion. Not only that, they should be practical, cheap and durable. Expensive machines are out of the question. Fortunately, we now have a vast wealth of fitness toys to choose from. You can make some of these toys on your own or you can purchase them through functional fitness suppliers.

medicine balls

Free weights have long been favored by functional trainers because they mimic the actual physical characteristics of common real-world objects. Boxes, grocery bags, building materials and small children are all "free," untethered objects. Medicine balls are also free weights, but have the additional advantage that we can throw, pass, roll and bounce them. Medicine balls are now manufactured in a vast range of sizes and textures so their use is basically unlimited. Some are lightweight and are ideal for challenging delicate muscles such as the rotator cuff of the shoulder. Others bounce and can be integrated into all sorts of games. Some of them float and make great pool games.

In general, the classic use of the medicine ball is for core body conditioning and core body games. Throwing a heavy ball demands participation by the hips and abdominals, which is exactly what we're looking for. Be sure to emphasize diagonal, cross-body movements that engage your abdominals. Make it a game and you're on your way.

physioball

The physioball is sometimes called a Swiss ball. If you haven't seen one, they're just like beach balls, except that manufacturers now make them with thick, burst-resistant walls which makes them ideal for a wide range of games and exercises.

Most people use the ball for stretching. This is a good beginning, but the number of possible ball movements is endless. The great thing about the physioball is that it is completely unstable. If you sit or lean on it, it's always trying to get away from you, which forces you to make constant adjustments; this in turn promotes physical

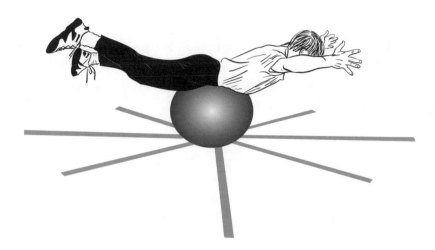

intelligence. Use this instability to your best advantage by inventing positions and movements that are right on the edge of what's possible.

The beauty of the physioball is that you can target your abdominals in many different ways. You can isolate or integrate. You can emphasize strength, flexibility or posture. You can add dumbbells or medicine balls to the mix and create dozens of games. In any case, look for ways to challenge your body core. Don't overlook the hard-core possibilities either. If you're inclined towards elite functional strength training, you can do killer sets of dumbbell lifts on the ball in a variety of positions.

jump ropes

Jump ropes are simple, cheap and consistently underrated. Not only are there lots of possible stepping, skipping and cross-over combinations, but you can also experiment with different ropes. The slender leather rope favored by boxers is good for speed training, but you can also get a heavy rope for a powerful pump.

hula hoops

Not just for doing the hula, these rings are incredibly versatile. Use them as targets for medicine ball passing games or for quick hop-scotch type games. Hula hoops are also essential for the notorious med ball slam-dunk.

cones and stepping hurdles

Cones and low hurdles are cheap, indestructible and you can arrange them in thousands of combinations. Slalom around cones. Run, jump and hop over hurdles. Place them wide for an endurance challenge, narrow for speed and agility.

stretch cord

Stretch cords are cheap, simple, adaptable and available in a variety of weights. Every trainer has a set of recommended stretch cord exercises, but the fact is that you can create whatever movements you like. You can play with hundreds of possible joint angles, speeds and ranges of motion.

Stretch cords are ideal for traveling as well. Put a few in your carry-on bag and when you get to your hotel room set 'em up however you like. Tie one to the door knob or a bed frame and you're ready to go.

Stretch cords are extremely useful in rehabilitation because you can start with very light resistance and do lots of reps. Then, as your strength increases, you can move on to thicker cords and then to free weights. In advanced athletic training, use the stretch cord in conjunction with the wobble board to increase the challenge. You'll soon find that the easiest shoulder rotation becomes a significant challenge.

the wobble board

The wobble board is a simple disk with a hemispherical form on the underside. Commonly used to rehabilitate ankle sprains and other injuries of the knee and hip, it is becoming increasingly popular in athletic training rooms. It is one of the all-time greatest exercise toys.

The wobble board is therapeutically valuable because it forces the patient to use his sensory and motor nervous system in a highly functional manner. Most people would call it a balance challenge, but we could just as well describe it as a sensory-motor challenge.

The wobble board is great fun, but it's misleading to think of it exclusively as a toy. In fact, the wobble board is just a natural extension of our bipedal anatomy. If you look at the shape of the bones in your hips and legs, this will become obvious. The hip joint, for example, is a true ball and socket. The heel bone (calcaneous) is very close to being spherical and the knee joint surfaces, while not spherical, are highly unstable as well. So, when we stand on the wobble board, we're really just amplifying a physical characteristic that already exists. This makes it an ideal functional training device.

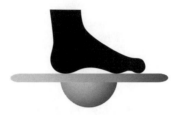

The basic challenge begins with simply trying to stand on the board. Try it on one foot; this is more functional because it mimics your normal walking challenge. Once you've mastered that, you can try any number of multi-plane movements. Try reaching to the points of the compass rose, high and low.

For maximum functionality, practice stepping on and off the board, just as you might step on or off a loose rock or patch of mossy ground on the trail. The ability to stand motionless on the board is interesting, but the real payoff comes when you can translate your wobble board skills into real-world locomotion challenges.

Then, once you feel comfortable with these basic movements, you can go wild. Stand on the wobble board and pass a medicine ball back and forth, for example. Even better, set up a series of boards and practice stepping from one to the next, just as you would cross a stream on a series of slippery rocks.

Creating the right conditions for play

The best gymnastic exercises of all are those which
not only exercise the body but also bring delight
to the mind.

Galen

If we're going to promote play, we're going to have to understand
how to create the right conditions. While play is often spontaneous, it's also the case that we can improve the odds if we set up the
right environment and circumstances. This is something that we
can do intentionally.

The first consideration is physical safety. Obviously, animals need
to feel safe and relatively secure before play can begin. If the creature
is concerned about injury or danger–real or imagined–play will be
inhibited. A common concern among would-be exercisers is the fear
of physical injury. People don't play because they don't want to hurt
themselves. Older bodies are not as resilient, especially if they've
been on the couch for several years. In many cases, this fear of injury
is fully justified.

There are a couple of ways that we can ease this inhibition and
promote play. First, we need to provide play environments that
are clean, orderly, well-maintained and reasonably safe. More importantly, we need to empower individuals to exercise their own
judgment in adjusting their level of participation. The programs that
we create must be flexible and individuals must be encouraged to
modify their movements according to their capabilities. This must
be made explicit. Too many programs force participants–either
overtly or covertly–to perform at a certain level. Peer pressure is
brought to bear on anyone who slacks off.

This is strictly an old-school approach. Physical education, if it is
anything, is about discovering what works for your body. To put it

another way, we can say that physical intelligence is as much about judgment as it is about lean body mass or aerobic capacity. When we play, we're learning to push the envelope, but we should also be learning how to adjust our intensity—easing up if necessary, modifying the quality of our movements or stopping altogether.

Not only do we need to give students permission to adjust their participation in movement, we should build this in as a foundational educational objective. That is, we should be teaching one another how to adjust the quality and quantity of our movement. Instead of creating an exercise culture that honors people who "play in pain" and continually pushes people to the brink, we ought to be more sophisticated. Our respect and admiration should go, not to those who "exceed the limits," but to those who exercise good physical judgment. If we honor intelligence in physical activity, people will be more likely to participate.

social inhibition

Physical danger inhibits many of us to be sure, but the thing we need to remember is that danger need not be real, only perceived. From the brain's point of view, it makes no difference whether the threat actually exists or if it is simply the product of the imagination; if you're afraid, you're less likely to play.

We can see this clearly when we look at the atrophy of play that often comes in adulthood. Children have no inhibitions about play; they just do it. Sometime later, the situation reverses itself. Adults, overwhelmed by work and convinced of the value of discipline, narrow their focus and play less frequently. We create, but we often hit plateaus or go stale. After a time, our physical comfort zone begins to contract.

Vigorous play would expand our physical repertoire and give us a renewed sense of vitality, but we are reluctant. In a great many cases, we avoid physical play because we feel inhibited by the watchful eyes of others. Afraid of looking foolish, we stick to movements and activities that we're familiar with. Secretly, we may want to go wild with exuberant, joyful movement, but the fear of public exposure holds us back.

Our inhibition to physical play is quite similar to our inhibition over singing, dancing or doing creative art in public. It is also related to our intense fear of public speaking. We've learned to dislike exposure. We're so accustomed to being judged and evaluated by our peers that we are reluctant to expose ourselves further unless we are highly adept at what we're doing. If we are beginners or only marginally competent, we prefer to hide out.

This is yet another reason to de-emphasize competition when possible. Being social animals, we are already programmed for high levels of sensitivity to public review. By creating a culture of competitive relationships, we ratchet up the pressure even higher.

What we really need here is permission to make fools of ourselves in public settings. Perhaps if we were more tolerant of one another, we might see more singing, dancing, art and play in public settings. This is an approach that we can build into exercise programs and into our fitness culture as a whole. Instead of worshipping the technical perfection of highlight clip, we'd do better if we simply concentrated our attention on having a good time.

This is something Jackie Chan teaches us in his movies. Obviously, he has expert movement skills, but his real genius lies in his playful spirit and his willingness to expose himself. The outtakes and bloopers at the end of his movies are not only fun, they are also inspirational. If Chan feels free to expose himself, so should we.

freedom from rank

Unfortunately, as a culture, we do a terrible job of creating environments and conditions that allow for playful behavior. In both school and work, ever-tightening performance standards squeeze us from every direction. We are asked to account for and document more and more of what we do. And in schools, the tyranny of sporting achievement chokes off play even before children are out of grade school.

A better solution is to offer participants some freedom from evaluation. This is not to say that we should toss out all performance standards and give free reign to all our physical impulses. Rather, we should offer opportunities for play that are socially safe.

One reason that play is so commonly undervalued is that it doesn't contribute to our dominance hierarchies. Success in play is entirely subjective; only you can say whether your last play session was pleasurable. Because play is subjective, it can't be measured and since it can't be measured, it can't be used to create rankings.

Hard-core rankists dismiss play because it can't contribute to a dominance hierarchy. But this is precisely why play is so valuable. Free from the incessant, dominating grind of measurement and comparison, participants can actually concentrate on the quality of their experience.

We are so conditioned to creating rank and hierarchy that we rarely stop to ask why we're doing it. It's reflexive. Assemble a group of social animals and it won't be long before someone comes up with a measurement and ranking system and begins to inflict it on everyone else. We do this obsessively with physical education and sport. Our default behavioral program says, "when in doubt, measure something and set up a ranking system."

While some people thrive in a rank-oriented environment, many people find it stifling and intimidating. The prospect of compulsory evaluation drives many would-be participants away. This is especially true in the world of exercise, where many people feel insecure about their bodies to begin with. And besides that, many of us are forced to endure relentless ranking pressures on the job each day. We are constantly being scrutinized, judged, labeled, evaluated and pigeon-holed. The last thing we need in our exercise programs is more of the same.

correct form kills play

When seeking to promote play, it's important to recognize other forces and orientations that inhibit what we're trying to do. One of the most notorious is the cult of "correct form."

If you make the rounds in today's fitness culture, you're likely to hear exercisers boasting about having "good form." You'll also hear personal trainers instruct their students to "maintain correct form" in their exercises. This advice has become ubiquitous, in spite of the fact that there is little evidence to demonstrate that it actually means anything. When we hear individuals talk about "correct form," we tend to assume that this knowledge is the result of some great biomechanical truth that has been verified in a laboratory or proven in clinical trials. In fact, there is little consensus among experts as to what constitutes "correct form" in any exercise. Most of what we believe on this subject comes from simple tradition.

Now obviously, there are some gross movement distortions that we would do well to avoid. Yes, if you're lifting a heavy weight, you'll probably do better if you engage the big muscles of your legs, hips and torso rather than simply jerking the weight off the floor with your upper body. Yes, if you're doing lunges, your knees will surely be a lot happier if you don't push them way out over your toes. But beyond that, "correct form" is mostly what works for you; if your movement is smooth, agile, powerful and enjoyable, it's probably correct.

Not only is the claim to universally correct movement form largely without foundation, it also tends to stifle physical play. Paradoxically, advocates of correct form end up inhibiting the very thing that they are trying to promote–frequent, vigorous and exuberant movement. Afraid that they might be violating some esoteric biomechanical principle, many would-be exercisers quit before they even begin. Intimidated by the notion that physical movement is a mind-bending branch of neuromuscular, biomechanical computation, beginners choose the couch instead. This orientation leads directly to one of the most popular excuses now in vogue with the exercise-avoidant. "I can't afford to hire a personal trainer and I don't want to move the wrong way and hurt myself, so I'm not going to start. Can't be too careful, you know."

In fact, non-human animals have been playing, hunting and fleeing for millions of years without the slightest bit of instruction in correct form. They don't know anything about biomechanically optimal movements; they simply follow the impulses provided by their nervous systems. They chase, pursue, dodge, evade and roll in the grass; all completely without knowledge of correct form. Obviously, such knowledge is not essential to survival.

"Correct form" fanatics will continue to push their agenda, of course, but we can refute their dogma with a single name: Dick Fosbury. Fosbury, as you may recall, broke with "correct form" and jumped over the high bar backwards. His coaches may have been appalled at such blatant violation of accepted norms and expert advice, but nevertheless, this "incorrect form" led directly to a long string of world records and is now the only method used by elite high jumpers.

Stoking the fire

The best climber is the one who has the most fun.

commonly-ignored climbing axiom

When we play, we're excited and enthusiastic. There's no labor involved, no drudgery. We're focused, engaged and attentive. In other words, we're stoked.

This terminology, of course, comes to us from the lexicon of surfing. The informal definition is "to be exhilarated, excited or euphoric, usually as the result of riding big waves." Classically, the surfer comes back to the beach after a good ride on a big wave and tells his friends "I was totally stoked." Over the years, "being stoked" has come to mean someone's enthusiasm for their sport and for life in general.

I use this term, not just because I happen to like it, but because there is no other word that so richly describes this fundamental aspect of play. In the serious adult world, the word "stoked" is dismissed as slang, part of the youth culture and thus unworthy of serious consideration. Actually, the art and practice of being stoked is fundamental to human function and happiness; it ought to be the object of serious investigation and studied at the highest levels.

What exactly does it mean to be stoked? Surely there is some special brain chemistry at work here, but being stoked is not simply a state of neurochemical excitation. A double espresso might jump-start your fire, but no amount of caffeine will substitute for genuine passion. Some people will no doubt suggest that being stoked is a state of synchrony between the body's nervous, endocrine and digestive systems, but there's more to being stoked than mere physiological efficiency. Being stoked is a whole body-mind-spirit engagement with life.

Naturally, there is tremendous variability in the nature of an individual's enthusiasm and engagement. What lights my fire might very well throw water on yours. (As the climber's bumper sticker says, "My best vacation is your worst nightmare.") Nevertheless, there are some common qualities that we see in every case.

When we're stoked, we're in the midst of a positive feedback loop of creative action and reinforcing sensation. The more we commit ourselves to the process, the better it feels. The reward comes, not from the feeling you get at the end, but in the quality of experience you get along the way.

In all cases, being stoked is an active pursuit of experience. It is pro-active and positive. Being stoked is never about running away from something. Rather, it comes from an active seeking and outward embrace, a fascination and love for some process, some experience. Being stoked is about desire, passion, longing, not about fear or denial. When you're stoked about movement and exercise, you're not fleeing in panic from fat, old age or heart disease, you're running towards agility, strength, endurance and new possibilities for play. You're running towards powerful movement, vitality, competence and functionality.

Being stoked assumes participation, immersion and engagement. The greater your sense of involvement, the hotter the burn. Yes, you can get temporarily stoked as a spectator, hanging on to the fate of your favorite sports team, but being a fan can only keep the fire burning for so long. You cannot build or intensify your stoke at arm's length; you cannot phone it in. You have to show up and put your body on the line.

Naturally, there is risk involved. The stoked experience is characterized by promise and surprise. As you stand on the beach looking out at the huge sets rolling in, you're tantalized by the possibility that you might actually be able to ride one. It's also a function of your curiosity. I wonder if I could ride that wave, run that hill, dunk that ball, lift that weight or swim that lake. There's no guaranteed outcome here, only possibility.

Significantly, there is a strong consensual agreement in the surfing community that, in the context of living well, being stoked is far more important than technical ability. Enthusiastic engagement is what it's all about. Who cares if you can't handle that gently breaking 3 foot roller? If you're loving the process, you're doing it right, even if you're getting pounded into the beach with every ride. This, of course, runs absolutely counter to our highlight-clip sport culture in which execution is considered the highest good. It also explains why many surfing and skateboard activists are trying to keep Nike out of their sport; such influence would inevitably distort the core values.

It's tempting to assume that being stoked is synonymous with the "peak experience" that we often hear about in the context of athletic competition. This is a mistake however because being stoked is really about the totality of the process. In fact, focusing exclusively on the peaks can distract us from the complete experience and cause it to break down.

In order to have an authentic stoke, you must be equally engaged across the whole enterprise. If surfing, you can't just be stoked about good waves on good days with good friends. You must also be stoked about cold, flat and foggy days when your friends have left and gone back to work. Similarly, we can't just be stoked about those peak exercise days when we set personal records, hoist big weights or beat the daylights out of the competition. And, even more to the point, we can't just limit our enthusiasm to those days when the scale and the tape measure tell us that we've lost weight.

Being stoked is about loving the totality of the process—not just the days when you feel light, agile and strong, but the bad days too, when you feel sore, slow and flabby. The process cycles and will always do so. It's OK to hate the really bad parts, the days when you get dragged across the coral on an undertow—just so long as you love it all.

The authentic stoke is always intrinsically motivated, powered by the individual's own passion. Yes, we can draw motivation from outside sources, including the enthusiasm of our friends and playmates. And we can draw some fire by watching the outlandish feats of professional athletes at their best. But in the end, it has to be our own desire that moves us.

ignition sources

Getting stoked may sometimes be a case of fortuitous inspiration, but it is not necessarily an accident either. You might get lucky and stumble into the right circumstances that light your fire. You can't force yourself into a stoke by an act of will but you can position yourself for optimum exposure to the possibility.

Curiosity lights the fire and keeps it going even in the face of strong winds and downpours. The stoked animal asks, What is it? How does it work? I wonder if I could do that? Inquisitiveness is at the root of the inferno. As soon as you stop asking questions, the curiosity wanes and your the fire fades.

Another great source of fuel is the enthusiasm of other people; a good stoke is contagious. Keep yourself stoked by spending time with other people who are similarly excited about their lives and movement. Ideally, you'll find a partner who is stoked on functional exercise and play, but in fact, any fire is contagious. Choose your friends for their fire and their spunk. Maybe you're not interested in astrophysics, orchestral music or island biogeography, but if you meet people who are really passionate about these things, some of their heat is bound to rub off. Find yourself some well-stoked role models and listen to their stories.

sustainability

What we're looking for here is not just a temporary charge that gets us up off the couch. We're trying to create a pattern of consistent movement, powered by imagination. We're looking for something sustainable.

If you're not stoked about what you're doing, maybe your body is trying to tell you something. You've probably exhausted the current object of your attention and you need to move on to some other level. Maybe you're overtraining. Or, it just might be the case that you're not paying attention to the possibilities. A lack of heat is a failure of curiosity, a failure of imagination. The way to increase your stroke is to feed your sense of wonder.

The problem comes on the day when we wake up and realize that we just don't want to make the plunge into the water or do another workout at the gym; oddly, we realize that we just aren't stoked.

Maybe the water has been too cold, the waves are flat and you're out of money and your partner has split for the world of salaries and comfort. On days like these, you can hardly manage a spark, much less a fully stoked blaze of desire and passion. And everyone, even the most perpetually stoked among us, has days like this. And yet, some of us rekindle the fire and get back in the water.

The difference lies in what we use as fuel. The poorly stoked among us can only run on one kind of fuel. The waves have to be a big, they've got to break to the left, the water has to be warm and the locals have to be friendly; otherwise, the fire dies out fast and fades into frustration. But the fully-stoked personality can burn just about anything for fuel; here we find the experiential omnivore. Sure, the waves are flat and the locals are hostile, but check out these fish! And those birds! And isn't there a place where we can go to dive off the cliffs? And I've been itching to take some underwater photos.

And so it goes for the fully stoked exerciser. Yes, your knee hurts and you can't go outside because the weather is really bad, but there's a new climbing gym in town that we could check out. And there's some cool new moves we can do on the physioball. And I'll bet if we played around a little, we could figure out how to do a really killer upper body workout right here at home.

GoAnimal games

There are lots of ways to have fun with primal movement challenges. With a little imagination, you'll be able to come up with ways to mimic ancestral conditions that are appropriate for your participants and location. Here are a few ideas to get you started.

Carnivore!

This is a field game with a superficial resemblance to Capture the Flag or Sharks and Minnows. Use a huge field if possible, preferably a mosaic, semi-wooded grassland park. (Actually, a major National Park would be ideal.) Assemble your participants and assign roles to each player: either hominid or carnivore. You can adjust the ratio as you see fit, but I have found that a good ratio is one predator for every 4 or 5 hominids. The idea is to keep the uncertainty high by spreading the predators out over the landscape.

Next, set up the predators with some sort of identification; a baseball cap or distinctive T-shirt would be a good choice, or use a predator mask if you can get one. Dispatch the predators out onto the playing field and direct them to lay low. They can work in small groups or solo, depending on their designated species and disposition.

Now send the hominids on a mission across the park. Their objective is to get across the open field to an imaginary lush, fertile valley on the other side. Give them a landmark to shoot for, a safe haven.

When the game begins, the hominids set out at whatever pace they choose. They may travel in groups or if they are really brave, solo. In any case, they will soon be vulnerable; they may be set upon by a carnivore at any time.

To score a "bite," a carnivore must land a distinct hand touch on the hominid's torso. Make this a judgment call on the honor system. If the touch is solid, the carnivore has won and the hominid drops out of the game. If it's a glancing touch, the hominid can continue, although he might consider himself injured. Any hominids who make it to the safe haven can declare victory for the day.

If you choose, you can make the game more compelling by training the carnivores to behave in a realistic fashion. That is, avoid long-distance running chases that drag on for miles; these simply test the endurance of one human against another. Instead, the predator should sprint at high speed and exhaust fairly quickly. This gives the hominid a more authentic experience.

You can also keep a more definitive score by using chalk. Set up each predator with a climber's chalk bag and outfit the hominids with dark-colored T-shirts. When the hominids ultimately arrive at the safe haven, the results should be obvious. If your shirt is covered with hand-prints, you can assume that you have been consumed.

This game is valuable because it rewards a diversity of skills. The fastest runner is not necessarily the survivor. A hominid might make it to the safe haven because of his agility, alertness, navigation, peripheral vision, social positioning or just plain wits. Similarly, the fastest carnivore won't score the most "bites" either. Timing, stealth and agility are just as important as speed.

Ideally, this game will not be played as a stand-alone activity. An innovative teacher can create an integrated approach, with classroom lectures, reading and homework all meshing with the physical game. Students could learn about biology, grassland ecology, human origins and evolution. The more comprehensive the approach, the more meaningful the game.

bucket brigade

This game uses medicine balls and 2 hula hoops. Set the hula hoops on opposite sides of the room or play area. You can adjust the distance to suit your needs. Put an equal number of medicine balls in each hoop. Now set up two teams or make it a head-to-head competition. In either case, the object of the game is simple; try to empty your hoop and fill up your competitor's hoop before he fills up yours.

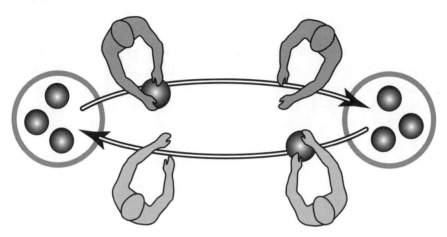

The possibilities for movement between the hoops are just about endless. You can run with the ball or pass it between team-mates. You can add obstacles or diversions. You can place the hoops really close together to emphasize speed, or you can place them far apart for a more sustained, pumpy workout. You can hop or lunge-walk with the ball or you can run over hurdles.

In any case, the game proceeds until there is a clear winner or until the system breaks down in general hilarity–a fairly common occurrence. Medicine balls are ideal for this game, but you can also find workable substitutes.

slam dunk with med balls and hula hoops

If you're looking to burn off lots of energy, this is a great way to go. All you really need is one med ball and one hula hoop. The hoop master holds the hoop at an appropriate height and the athlete simply starts throwing it down. Of course, as soon as you've slammed the ball through the hoop, you'll have to chase it down, pick it up and run back to the hoop. But the hoop master, devious trainer that he is, will have moved to a new location, forcing you to swerve, change directions and adjust. If you like, you can count the number of dunks per minute or you can just go until you start getting sloppy. If you're the hoop master, be sure to heckle your player and keep him moving strong.

med ball pass through hula hoop

This game is highly dynamic. Start out in pairs with simple passing back and forth. A medicine ball is ideal here, but you could also use a basketball or volleyball. When the participants are warmed up, set up in groups of three. One person acts as the hoop master, holding the hoop vertically between the participants. The objective is to pass the ball through the hoop to your partner.

If the hoop master just stood still, this would be no great challenge, but instead, he moves erratically around the room, forcing the participants to continually adjust both their throws and their catches. You never know where the hoop is going to be next, so you'll have to be ready to change direction. The hoop master makes or breaks this game. The trick is to be slightly unpredictable and erratic to force good movement, but not so radical as to make it impossible. Go until someone drops the ball, then switch partners.

rope-a-dope

This is a full body game that will test your stability, proprioception and cunning. Get yourself a rope about 10 feet long and square off with your partner. Each person will grab the rope at about the one third position; this leaves about 3 feet of rope between you and your partner. You can grab the rope with either hand or both, it makes no difference.

Now stand on one foot. The object of the game is to get your partner off balance. If you hop or step down with the other foot, you're out and you'll have to start over. The basic strategy is to use some combination of pulling—as in tug of war—and letting slack slide through your hands. This makes it a yin-yang challenge.

Obviously, you can only do the slide trick so many times before you run out of rope, so you'll have to be wary; if you let the rope slide to the end, you'll run out of options. Similarly, you should try

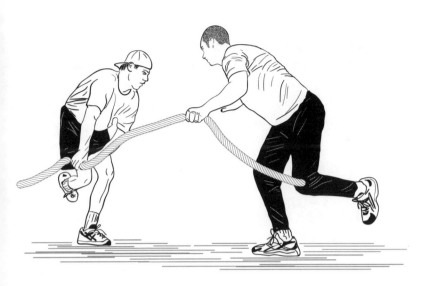

to reel in slack whenever you can; it will give you an advantage. As you will soon discover, strength doesn't help much in this game; speed, abdominal function and whole-body coordination makes the difference. Be sure to switch partners frequently. Everyone seems to have their own strategy and surprises. You can also create variations; standing side-to-side or even back-to-back for example.

king of the circle

This game is simple. Just set up a circle roughly six to eight feet in diameter. (Lay down a rope or mark the circle with tape.) Step inside the circle with your partner and put your hands behind your back. Now, try to push or sucker your partner out of the circle. Use your hips and shoulders as primary points of contact.

The challenge will become instantly obvious; if you push too hard and your partner spins or side-steps, you'll be out. Conversely, if you're too soft and squishy, you'll get pushed out. You'll need to be both strong and flexible, stable and mobile.

This game works well with a group. Start with a pair of people in the circle. When someone gets pushed out, a fresh person cycles right in to keep the game going. You'll be amazed at how much this one pumps your legs. If the participants get too amped and competitive, you may need to tone it down a bit; instruct people to use a little less power and a little more skill.

This game is not only fun, it is highly appropriate for martial art and general combative training. It's like judo without arms, and you'll learn the same skills, sensitivity and the physical judgment that tells you when to be strong and when to be soft.

Integration:
putting it all together

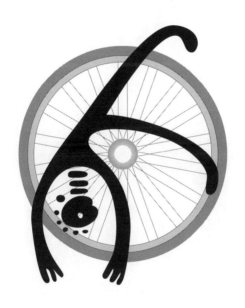

The cyclic path to skill and fitness

In conventional exercise programs, we are used to thinking about fitness in terms of calories, heart rates, lactic acid, aerobics, weight training and stretching. These are certainly elements of the process, but if we really want to get down to the fundamentals, we're going to have to talk about the rhythms of our physical experience, the waves and oscillations of training intensity and volume. As it turns out, the way we manage this oscillation will be crucial to our success.

the variables: frequency and amplitude

Any wave or oscillation can be described with two simple variables. On one hand we can talk about the height or amplitude of the wave. In fitness training, amplitude is a measure of the intensity or volume of the physical challenge. A series of hard, vigorous workouts forms a high amplitude wave; a series of easy workouts is low amplitude.

When we adjust the amplitude of our training programs, we make changes in the intensity of the challenge. There are several key points to keep in mind here. First, high amplitude is good; intensity stimulates the body. If all the other variables are equal, high-effort training tends to give us the best performance results. If you shock the body with physical challenge, it will attempt to supercompensate as specifically as possible for the microscopic injury that you've inflicted.

We can also talk about the wave's frequency; this refers to how often we're training. If you're working out twice a day, your training wave is high-frequency. If you're working out once a month, your wave is low frequency. Naturally, we can adjust these two variables in many possible combinations; low-low, high-high, high-low and low-high for example.

When we ask questions about training frequency, we're asking questions like "How often should I work out?" Of course, every fitness expert has some universal formula that we're supposed to follow, but the fact remains that everyone is different and even if we had identical bodies, our physical objectives are different. Consequently, there can be no universal formula for training frequency.

We do know that some measure of repetition is essential. If you only apply the stimulus once, the body has no chance to recognize a pattern and thus has no motivation to supercompensate. One big run might make you feel good on that particular day, but if that's all you do this year, your body won't be stimulated to create much of a response. Similarly, if you apply the stimulus chaotically or randomly, your body will be in a constant state of confusion and your adaptations will be weak at best. Thus, some degree of regularity is essential.

Since the body generates tissue adaptation in response to periodic challenge, it soon becomes obvious that adjusting the amplitude and frequency of the program is critical to success. Adjustments to these two variables can make or break a training program. This is why we now see coaches and trainers obsessing over seasonal cycles, macrocycles, microcycles and mesocycles, all under the name "periodization." The details can get amazingly subtle, but the game is always the same, to adjust the oscillations between physical challenge and rest.

common errors

When we look at oscillations in fitness training, we see a couple of common themes. First are errors of amplitude. The most common, of course, is the error of low-amplitude. Low amplitude exercisers never break a sweat. They like the idea of vigorous movement, but only in the abstract. Gentle movement without striving is of course far better than nothing, but the payoff will be minimal.

Errors of high amplitude are not as common, but are not unusual either, especially in hyper-competitive sporting environments. Major athletic events can be extremely high-amplitude and can extract a tremendous physiological toll. Naturally, it makes sense to assume that a high-amplitude challenge should be matched by an equal and opposite measure of high-amplitude rest.

Then we have errors of frequency. Obviously, low-frequency is a common theme in today's world. These exercisers challenge themselves, but fail to do it frequently enough to stimulate a physiological response. If you do a good session of weight lifting and then take a few weeks off, you'll just wind up getting sore; the body assumes that the challenge was a singular event, not something to pay much attention to.

Errors of high-frequency are actually pretty common, particularly among highly-motivated physical achievers; not a day goes by without some sort of physical push. If this gives pleasure, there can be no arguing with it, but for many people, such high-frequency doesn't really allow adequate time for healing, nor is it truly necessary for health. A professional athlete may need to train nearly every day, but that is a specialized physical application. The rest of us will do better with regular days off.

Another common error is sheer randomness. Instead of adhering to a fairly regular cycle, many amateurs bounce from one physical activity to another; amplitude and frequency are in a constant state of flux. Dabblers train hard one week, slack off for two, then shift to an entirely different sort of physical challenge. The body is constantly trying to find some consistent stress pattern to adapt to, but none exists. This problem afflicts many modern people, simply because it is often difficult to maintain any kind of physical regularity in the face of today's chaotic challenges.

Surprisingly, the other common error is to practice an oscillation that is excessively regular and overly patterned. This is the Monday-Wednesday-Friday syndrome. It is not unusual to meet people in the gym who have been doing precisely the same routine for years, even decades. Back and biceps one day, chest and triceps the next, legs and abs on the third day. If it's Monday, I must be doing curls.

The problem here is that the body adapts to the stimulus, usually after about 6 weeks. If you continue with the same oscillating pattern, your body will have less and less motivation to adapt. You'll be maintaining health, but you won't be making much progress in performance. The solution is to introduce variations into your routine, modifications to speed, resistance, reps or sets. This is where play also becomes extremely valuable. Since play is inherently diverse, the body will be stimulated towards further adaptation.

The other common error is the failure to make the training oscillation progressive. Here we see exercisers who select a work-out program and then jump right in at full-intensity, right off the couch. This leaves them sore and possibly injured. A better approach is to establish a progressive, tapered oscillation that starts out with low amplitude. Gradually, over the course of several weeks, increase the amplitude and possibly the frequency as well. This requires some degree of foresight, restraint and discipline. You may have to keep your enthusiasm in check for awhile and allow your physiology to catch up with what you want to do. Take your time.

raise your intensity and volume in a cyclic, progressive fashion
ease into it - train hard, then rest - then train even harder

musicians and scholars

In setting up an oscillating pattern for physical education and fitness, we can take some practical instruction from the experts in nervous system training, the musicians and the scholars. Remember, physical fitness is about more than just muscle and adipose tissue; the way we train the nervous system is crucial to our success.

In music, the recommended formula has been pretty well worked out by now. Most music teachers advise students to practice frequently, in short, highly-focused sessions. The idea here is that the student should pump his or her nervous system with high-frequency, high-amplitude practice sessions. Don't do endless repetitions of scales and chords; concentrate hard, then quit and come back to it later. Yes, we sometimes hear about musicians who get so immersed in what they're doing that they play for 8 hours at a stretch, but this is usually the advanced student who manages to tap into a personal power source. Beginners are advised to stick to the short-session formula.

Educators and test-taking experts advise the same pattern for academic preparation. It is folly to put in an all-nighter before the final exam; spread out your efforts over frequent, short and highly-focused sessions. If you're trying to prepare for a dreaded SAT, LSAT or bar exam, set up a pattern of regular oscillation; study hard for an hour or so, then play or sleep. As every serious student knows, it makes little sense to slack off all quarter and then cram the night before the exam. Instead, grow your nervous system function and information processing abilities with short, intense study periods alternating with quality rest. In this, the scholar and the athlete are united in the same quest.

high-contrast living

Naturally, the way you set up your training oscillation will depend on what you're trying to accomplish. If all you're after is basic health, you don't need super-high amplitude or frequency. You don't even need clockwork regularity. For basic health, any fairly regular pattern of moderate challenge and rest works pretty well. There's a pretty big window here; as long as your lifestyle includes regular vigorous movement, you're going to enjoy health benefits.

If, on the other hand, you want to excel at some particular sport or movement specialty, you'll want to experience high-amplitude challenges at the highest possible frequency. If you're really serious about making dramatic tissue changes, you'll want to stress your body as deeply as possible as often as you can. Obviously, this puts you at risk for overtraining because you'll be right up against the limit of your recovery ability; this becomes a race between physiology and catastrophe. If you attempt to sustain a high-amplitude, high-frequency program for too long, you'll probably find yourself getting injured.

In any case, the key to success in therapeutic oscillation is depth: hard training and deep rest. The deeper the cycling from challenge to rest, the better the result. Unfortunately, many of us have ex-

tremely shallow training cycles; we don't really challenge ourselves
and we don't really rest effectively either. We are flat-liners– working
fairly hard, taking it fairly easy.

What we really need for increased health and performance is an
increased pattern of contrast. Tony Yaniro, one of the finest rock
climbers of this generation, is a passionate advocate of this approach.
His advice for maximum performance is simple: "When you're
training hard, train really hard. When you're taking it easy, take it
really easy." In other words, create a high-contrast lifestyle. When
you train, push yourself like the devil. When you rest, power-lounge
like a professional beach bum.

It's easy to imagine that the life of the primal hominid was distinctly high-contrast. Hunting is hard work, especially when game
is scarce. You may have to push it really hard for a couple of days to
lay in a good supply of meat. Long distance travel, especially over
unfamiliar terrain can be exhausting. Add in some river crossings,
predator encounters and navigational errors and you've got a high-
amplitude physical challenge.

When you do make it back to camp, you're going to do what
comes naturally; that is, you're going to sit under a tree and relax.
And since there's no phone, fax or TV, you can really get down to
some serious, body-restoring leisure. Spend the day watching the
animals at the waterhole, chat with your tribe mates, nap, sing and
dance.

Paleolithic rhythm

As we have seen, an essential part of being a good animal is establishing a cycle of activity and rest that is appropriate for your species,
your age and the conditions you live in. Not only is this cyclic pattern a proven formula for athletic success, it also happens to match
precisely with the lifestyle of human hunter gatherers. Researchers
have documented this pattern by observing contemporary hunting
and gathering cultures such as the !Kung bushmen of Africa, and by
making deductions from fossil evidence.

In it's stripped-down simplicity, the pattern goes something like
this: The tribe leaves their temporary camp for two or three days of
highly vigorous overland travel that includes hunting, gathering and

fishing. This is a period of sustained movement and intense physical challenge. We've got our heart rates up for long periods of time, we're burning calories at a ferocious rate and we're pushing ourselves to cover lots of terrain. Upon returning to camp, the tribe enters a period of sleep, sloth, celebration and power-lounging. After a few days of leisure, we'll be hungry, curious or bored and we'll be setting out once again. In their book *The Pleistocene Prescription*, authors Eaton, Shostak and Konner called this pattern "The Paleolithic Rhythm." This cycle must have been repeated with variation millions of time throughout our history.

From a coach's point of view, the Paleolithic hunters and gatherers were following an ideal pattern for athletic excellence as well as general health. During their two to four day hunting outing, they pushed their bodies for strength and endurance. This caused significant microtrauma (sometimes macrotrauma!) to their tissues. Muscle cell membranes burst, capillaries exploded, nerve cells pumped their transmitters to exhaustion. Back at camp, their bodies not only repaired the damage, but laid down new and improved tissue in damaged areas, working under the assumption that such challenge was likely to be repeated. As this cycle was repeated over the course of months and years, hunters and gatherers would have made significant gains in strength and endurance, all without machines, supplements or spreadsheets.

We don't have to journey back to the Pleistocene to get a sense of the Paleolithic rhythm; we can simply observe our dogs. Take your pal on any kind of outdoor journey and he'll go wild, running and playing at high intensity for a day or maybe two. Then it's down time and deep sleep for a day or two. Then, if he can break free, it's back to another round of outdoor action. This cycle is fundamental to canine existence; it's no wonder that humans and dogs have lived together for so long. Professional dog trainers now advise owners to give their animals the chance to follow this kind of oscillation as much as possible. In fact, most of the behavior problems that dog owners suffer–barking, chewing, begging and general madness–can all be traced back to lack of exercise and failure to follow some sort of Paleolithic rhythm. And if such interruptions impact our dogs, we can be sure that we will suffer a similar fate with our own variations of barking, chewing, begging and general madness.

Some of the problems here are obvious. First, the 5, 6 or 7 day work week that we now endure bears no relationship to the Paleolithic rhythm or natural cycles of human physiology. Rather, it is a historical and cultural artifact that is now inflicted upon us and generally accepted without much protest. This is not some minor scheduling inconvenience however, but a serious challenge to every dimension of human health. By forcing us out of our natural physiological oscillation, the standard work week actually poses a significant health problem, one that we are all paying for, one way or another.

Perhaps, as society and business evolves, companies and institutions will restructure their schedules to be more humane and consistent with the natural cycles of human physiology. In the meantime, we're going to have to work with what we've got and adjust our cycles the best we can. We may not be able to control our obligatory labor, but we might be able to control the intensity, the amplitude and frequency of our optional activities.

Assertive creativity is the solution. If you can, try to cluster your physical challenges into discrete bursts that stretch over the course of a few days; then alternate with as much power-lounging as you can manage. You probably won't be able to push as hard or relax as deeply as your hominid ancestors, and you'll still have to fight off the myriad modern forces that will try to break your rhythm, but you might keep enough oscillation to stay healthy and happy.

The dose makes the difference

All things are poison and nothing is without poison.
It is the dose that makes a thing poisonous.

Paracelsus
16th century pharmacologist

We are accustomed to getting our fitness information from fitness professionals, so it will probably come as a surprise when I suggest that we take inspiration, if not outright instruction, from the field of toxicology. Toxicology is the study of poisons in biological systems. Typically, we think of poisons as substances that threaten the human body, but we can also take a broader view and study poisons in any system. We can look at poisons in lakes, rivers or the atmosphere for example.

Toxicologists have discovered a great deal about poisons at all levels, but their greatest discovery has to do with the crucial importance of quantity. As it turns out, no substance is inherently polluting or destructive; it just depends on how much there is in the system. Dioxins, DDT, saturated fat, nicotine–all obey the same law, regardless of the system. That is, the dose makes the poison. This law seems to hold true at just about any level of ecology or physiology you care to scrutinize. From drug and neurotransmitter concentrations in the human body, to alloy mixtures in metals, to dissolved gasses in alpine lakes–quantity makes the difference between success and failure, between health and illness. Ben Franklin would have agreed enthusiastically–the dose makes the tonic, the dose makes the poison.

The findings of toxicologists are routinely verified by our personal intuition and experience. Run a few miles a week and you'll enjoy a pleasant endorphin buzz and a healthy appetite; run a dozen miles every day and develop a lasting relationship with your physical therapist. Have one glass of wine and you'll feel a warm glow and sense of ease; have a whole bottle and you'll make a fool out of yourself. Quantity is key.

As for substances, so too for exercise. Common sense tells us that the perfect training quantity lies somewhere between sloth and fanaticism, between under-use and over-use, between inactivity and fitness heroics. Quantity is always key. The dose makes the poison, the dose makes the medicine.

the dose-response curve

When we think of the various challenges and substances that our bodies encounter in life, many of us tend to fall back on a simple explanation, the classic "common-sense" approach that says "if a little is good, more must be better." To put it in more technical language, we tend to think that the dose-response relationship is linear. Double the dose, double the payoff. Triple the dose, triple the payoff.

This kind of thinking is notorious in the world of exercise. They hyperactive fitness fanatic says, "If one hour of exercise is good, two hours must be twice as good." "If two sets of ten reps are good, then four sets of 20 reps must be four times as good."

As it turns out, this popular calculation is just plain wrong. We now know with complete certainty that the dose-response curve for exercise is not linear. Doubling the dose will not give you double the benefit. Tripling the dose will not give your triple the benefit. The dose-response curve for exercise is well, curved.

Consider a graph in which we compare exercise volume against physiological benefit. At the left end of the curve we find the minimal level of exercise, practiced by someone who is just a hair over absolute sedentary living. Let's say that he's been on the couch for the last few years and now decides that it's time to start moving. If this person goes for a short walk once a week, he'll enjoy a small measure of physiological benefit. If he doubles his frequency or intensity by walking twice a week, he'll probably double his benefit. If he triples and quadruples his volume, he'll enjoy a substantial physiological payoff.

This pattern will continue for some time, but at some point of volume, frequency and intensity, the curve will begin to level off and he'll have to work much harder to achieve any additional gains. But now let's suppose that he's not satisfied with his progress and decides to increase his training volume or intensity yet another notch. Now he's playing a risky game because sooner or later, the curve not only flattens out, it actually reverses in a downward direction. Further increases in volume, frequency or intensity will now result in a decrease in physiological payoff. In this zone, the harder you train, the worse you'll get. At this point, additional increases in exercise volume become, in the language of toxicology, poisonous.

The hot topic in many fitness publications these days is recognizing overtraining. Subtle symptoms include irritability, weight loss, poor sleep, lack of motivation and performance plateaus. Obvious symptoms include overuse injuries and performance downswings. If you are experiencing any of these symptoms, you'd do well to take another look at your exercise dosage. You may be on the wrong side of the dose-response curve. In other words, your body may be telling you to back off.

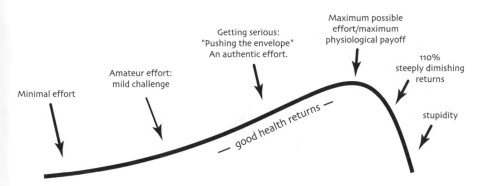

In any case, the important thing to notice about this curved relationship is that there is a pretty broad range for effective health promotion. You don't have to hit a specific intensity or frequency target with precision. Just about any level, from minimal (walking a few times each week) to semi-professional (hitting it hard on most days) will improve health. For most of today's sedentary folks, more is generally better, but there's a big window for effectiveness; as long as you're making a genuine, sincere effort, you don't have to follow a strict formula.

absolutism

This ecological principle of dose-dependency stands in marked contrast to the health care absolutism that is so popular today, the ideology that holds that some activities or substances are inherently bad: animal products, sugar, caffeine, take your pick. You can, if you choose, make a case for the destructive effects of each of these and you may even come up with a lot of supporting evidence, but the fact remains that any polluting effect of these substances will always depend on quantity, both in the short-term and the long term. As James Lovelock, the scientist behind "Gaia theory" put it, "Pollution is always about quantity."

Similarly, health care absolutism holds that some processes, experiences and substances are inherently virtuous regardless of quantity: brown rice, blue-green algae, tofu, yoga, weight-lifting, running—take your pick. But you can be sure that there is some upper limit to brown rice and tofu consumption; we can get too much of a good thing. It would be nice if we could live by simplistic rules, but the fact remains that we will always have to exercise judgments on quantity and quality.

in context

The important thing to remember is that finding the right level of movement is not simply a matter of fine-tuning your physiology. It's also about creating the kind of life that gives you satisfaction and meaning.

Yes, we can attempt to make the ideal quantities in a rational manner by taking measurements and noting the results. If we collect enough data and correlate it with outcomes we could, in theory at least, arrive at numbers for optimal quantities for things like exercise. But in many cases, especially in complex environments such as a human body, we're never going to have enough data to make the call. (How much red wine did they say was ideal for good health? Was it three glasses per week? Or six?)

The ideal quantity is not something that can be prescribed. Rather, it will always be a matter of individuality; individual genetics, personality, disposition and history. A good trainer, coach or therapist can inspire you to greater effort or help you make fine adjustments, but no one can tell you definitively the ideal number of reps, sets or mileage that is right for you. These are things that you must discover for yourself.

If we could input all the factors of our lives into one massive spreadsheet and run the numbers past a exercise scientist, we might, in theory, come up with a personalized formula for a balanced fitness program. But that's just not going to happen. In the first place, many parts of our lives simply cannot be quantified and besides, our objectives and our physiology is constantly in flux anyway. And since our lives are in flux, the ideal amount of movement we need for health is also in flux. This means that balance is not state but a process, not a point, but a path. Balance is not something we achieve, but something that we do. It's a game of constant adjustment.

Without some sort of conclusive data, we are left in the position of having to exercise some kind of personal, even aesthetic judgment. This means looking, not just for performance, but for beauty. And in this respect, integrating physical movement into our lives is nothing less than performance art.

The questions here are all about proportion. The numbers may look right, but what about the context? Yes, 50 miles per week just might be the ideal dose for increasing your VO_2 max and bringing your red blood cell counts up to their ideal levels. But if those 50 miles take away from another part of your life that deserves attention, you may just be creating a rather ugly piece of art.

Health stems directly from a appreciation of dose, scale, and proportion. Elements that are out of proportion tend to be ugly, whether they are too small or too big. In terms of physical fitness, exercise avoidance and exercise mania are both suspect.

Sure, there are probably some numbers out there in data land that would guarantee physical fitness excellence. But unless you are a professional athlete, these numbers must be balanced against competing interests and demands. The idea is to integrate movement into our lives, not abandon our lives for the sake of fitness.

Movement therapy

In the old days, everyone told us to rest when injured. If you sprained your ankle or wrenched your elbow, your doctor would have advised rest and may have even put the injured extremity in a cast. In fact, for a long time, the standard prescription for back pain was bed rest.

Today the trend is entirely different. Physicians and physical therapists now understand that movement actually accelerates the healing process and they encourage us to move injured body parts as soon as we can. Bed rest is no longer prescribed for back pain, for example. Far from being seen as a negative, the modern medical community now views movement as inherently therapeutic. Post-surgical rehab is a very active process; some patients in rehabilitation get more movement than at any other time in their lives.

Of course, not just any movement will enhance healing and get you back in action. It has to be the right kind of movement, executed with the right intensity, repeated at the right frequency. Ideally, we'd have the guidance of a physician or physical therapist every time we hurt ourselves, but in this day of diminishing medical resources, it's important to know something about basic rehabilitation so you can do some of it yourself. After all, if you're physically active, you're going to experience frequent, low-level injuries that don't really demand a trip to the clinic. If you have some strategies for basic rehabilitation, you'll get better faster and enjoy movement more completely.

prescription: high reps, low resistance

Obviously, you'll want to seek medical care for acute injuries. You'll also want to fight any inflammation with ice, anti-inflammatory medications and rest as necessary. Most amateur exercisers are familiar with these techniques by now.

Once you're starting to feel better, you can begin some passive movement. Technically, passive movement is simply movement without resistance, moving a limb or joint with no load whatsoever. In practice, it can get quite sophisticated.

You can either do it yourself or get someone else to help you. In any case, start by taking the joint through a conservative, comfortable range of motion. This will move fluid and keep the nervous system active. Massage the joint, shake it gently, roll it around; move it in several planes, several directions. Obviously, all of this has to be done without causing pain. Continue with passive motion for several days or as long as it takes to feel a reduction in pain. If it doesn't feel better, back off or see your physician.

Eventually, you should get to a stage where you're starting to feel more ambitious and eager for greater resistance. The typical prescription in this early-stage rehabilitation is to use high numbers of repetitions with low resistance. This makes good sense. The idea is to reap the therapeutic benefits of movement without overloading sensitive tissue.

You don't need weights or machines at this point. The weight of the injured limb itself may give you adequate resistance. Later, you can progress to small-diameter stretch cord. Do lots of reps and do sets frequently to maintain a high level of fluid turnover within the injured tissue. Later, you can increase the resistance with heavier stretch cord as you decrease the number of repetitions and the frequency of exercise. If pain begins to creep back in, decrease the resistance.

At this point, it is sometimes tempting to work the injured area directly by creating exercises that precisely mimic the original traumatic event or pattern. If something hurts, we reason, it must be weak. If it's weak, we need to strengthen it with exercise. There's a certain validity to this reasoning and it sometimes works, but it can also backfire into overtraining and overuse.

Sometimes, a more sophisticated strategy is to work indirectly. In many cases, the pain that we're experiencing is actually the result of weakness or slowness in some other part of the kinetic chain. Maybe the muscles of your hips aren't controlling the movement of your legs for example; the reason your knee hurts is that your butt isn't doing it's job. If you continue to work the muscles around your knee, you may not get anywhere. But if you start working above and below the injury, you might get better results.

In any case, you'll want to stress functional integration of your body. Get other muscles to share the load and protect weak tissue that's in the process of recovery. If something hurts, you might be able to get other muscles to participate in the chosen movement. The abdominals are a likely candidate.

change the frequency

Sometimes it's a traumatic event that gets us; you trip on a curb or fall off your bike. In these cases, it's pretty easy to identify the causal relationship between the original event and the pain that we feel. But in a disturbing number of cases, injuries seem to appear without apparent cause, out of the blue. We call these "over-use injuries" but that doesn't really explain very much. This kind of spontaneous pain is not only unsettling, it can be difficult to treat because we can't trace it back to an original trauma. Lots of active people get really upset and frustrated with these mysterious afflictions.

It may help to think about how these problems can come about over time. When you're exercising regularly, your body is constantly tearing itself down and building itself back up. In terms of physiology and muscle metabolism, we experience anabolic and catabolic processes constantly. Depending on what kind of condition you're in, the tissues of your body can tolerate a certain number of stress and rebuilding cycles in a given time period.

Let's suppose that, because of your genetics and training history, the tissues of your shoulder can tolerate say, 3 workouts per week or 12 cycles of stress per month. At this level of frequency you're doing fine, but let's say you want more out of your body and decide to add a couple of extra sessions to your schedule each month. At first, you probably won't notice any dramatic changes. But now your body is slowly falling behind in it's effort to maintain tissue integrity. The tissue in question is getting slightly weaker with each cycle and one day, weeks later, you wake up in pain. It wasn't any single event that got you, it was simply that your training frequency was too high for too long.

At this point you might be tempted to panic and go in search of specific therapies. Or, you might be tempted to stop your activity altogether. If the injury is minor however, a better approach might simply be to decrease the frequency of the challenge. If you simply do several fewer training sessions per month, your metabolism will eventually catch up. You'll still be able to maintain your overall health and activity-specific skills and, if you're patient, you'll get back to a pain-free condition.

injuries as opportunity

When we're injured, we're obviously looking for healing and we're trying to get back to the activities that give us pleasure and meaning. So we go in search of ice, anti-inflammatory medications and any other therapies that offer the promise of relief. Many of today's exercisers are well versed in the fundamentals of tissue rehab.

Knowing the physiology of healing is valuable, but we are also interested in the relationship we have with our injured bodies. In a sense, we're looking for a philosophy of injury. Since injury is very nearly inevitable in human life, it makes sense to consider what kind of meanings they hold for us.

For most of us, our relationship to injury is entirely adversarial. We curse our pain and the effect it has on our lives. Injuries compromise our performance and derail our plans. They interfere directly with the very thing that gives us pleasure and satisfaction. We wish the doctor could just give us a magic pill to make the pain go away. If the pain doesn't go away, we become irritable, grouchy and depressed.

Surely it makes sense to fight our pain and injury with whatever means modern medicine can provide us. Nevertheless, we can also do well by looking for the opportunities in our predicament. Unless the injury is extreme, this opportunity comes as pain forces us into new variations on familiar movements. Like it or not, you get to explore some variations and refinements.

For example, you might be able to adjust the amplitude of a favorite move, going a bit shallower or adding some rotation. Alternately, you might find that you can adjust the speed; a faster or slower movement might feel smoother or more coordinated. You might move more towards isolation or more towards integration. If you can spread out the loads by bringing in more muscles into the movement, that may give the injured tissues a chance to rest. Or, maybe you've just got a weak link that needs to be challenged.

In this way, pain and injuries can actually drive us towards physical creativity and intelligence. In the long run, minor injuries can actually be beneficial because they drive us towards adjustment and variation, in other words, skill. You're hurt, but you don't want to fester on the couch, so you begin to invent new movements that you can perform without pain. Maybe you can't do your favorite moves, but perhaps you can invent a fresh variation. When you finally do recover, you'll have a broader range of movement possibilities to play with.

More substantial injuries change the course of our lives and in the process drive us into new experience. Naturally, we resist this derailment, but we may also come to find the new experience stimulating and rewarding. And besides, who wants to do precisely the same movement pattern for their entire life?

Be an opportunist

Sensing that we need more movement in our lives, many of us go searching for some sort of regular exercise program. We want to get some regular exercise but unfortunately, our lives tend to be crazy, mixed up and sometimes out of control. Our schedules are changing all the time and just when we think that we've got all the loose ends nailed down, somebody throws a monkeywrench into the works. Entropy not only increases, it seems to actually accelerate.

Not surprisingly, one of the most common refrains from would-be exercisers is "I really need to get on a program." This phrase is uttered millions of times each day across America. In fact, one popular fitness book advises readers to *Get With the Program*. The sub-text implies that we need structure and external control. We talk as if we need some authority to regulate our behavior because, if left to our own devices, we will simply get distracted.

But, as we have seen, programs have largely failed to produce broad-based improvements in physical condition. Instead of more programs, we need to find a way to do what the Surgeon General has been saying all along. That is, we need to "weave physical activity into the fabric of our daily lives." We don't need something special, we need something ordinary. We don't need special events and organized structures, we need a style of living that includes movement.

The default program for the hunter-gatherer body says "Play when you like, move when you have to and rest whenever possible." As we have seen, this program worked on the grassland for several million years, but is generally inappropriate today. Somehow, we need to reprogram ourselves to a new orientation that says "Play when you like, work when you must and seize every opportunity for movement."

The trick, it seems, is to become an opportunist. Don't wait around for next organized exercise class; grab movement opportunities when they present themselves. If you get really good at this opportunistic approach, you might even find that you don't even need an "exercise program" at all. You'll become skilled at finding movement in unlikely situations and you'll eventually make a habit out of it.

For example, suppose you don't have time to exercise because you have to fly out of town on business. You're going to be stuffed into an airplane for several hours, but even being on an aircraft does not condemn you to complete stasis. Granted, short-haul flights in small aircraft are really tough, but on longer routes there's usually a little room to move around. You can stretch in the aisles, maybe even squeeze in a few lunges.

This approach is guaranteed to work; look for opportunities and you'll find dozens of ways to get some movement in your life without ever setting foot in a gym or going to a class. It's amazing how much movement you can sneak in when you're standing in line at the supermarket or the bank. Over the months and years, these efforts become medically significant. (A mere three minutes of movement per day over 30 years adds up to 550 hours of movement that you wouldn't get otherwise. Not enough for Olympic-caliber fitness, but far better than nothing.)

Suppose you need to make a big cross-country journey by car. You'll be cruising the interstate for a few days, so obviously you won't have the opportunity to exercise, or so it would seem. But along that interstate you'll notice that there are rest stops every 50 miles or so and you're probably going to stop to use the bathroom if nothing else. There's usually some comfortable shade at these rest areas, so let's suppose that every time you stop, you rally for a couple sets of lunges and a few push ups; maybe even toss a medicine ball around. No Olympian heroics here, no sweating, just a short movement session, then back into the car and away you go. By the time you get to your destination, you will have logged a couple of hundred reps and you'll probably feel pretty good too. Not bad for not having time to exercise.

Of course, most of us avoid these kinds of opportunistic behaviors because we are inhibited by the gaze of others; we don't want to attract attention in the departure lounge, the rest stop or the city park. If you start doing lunges at the rest area, people will look right at you. They might even point their fingers and whisper to each other; they might even shake their heads. You'll be labeled "deviant" or "eccentric."

The solution, as some have suggested, is that we must "be willing to be weird." Yes, that's a good start, and a philosophy that I certainly subscribe to, but then again, it's all a matter of perspective. That is, when we do vigorous movement in public, we are not the ones displaying aberrant behavior. We are normal animals; we are expressing our natural inclination to move when we feel like it. It's the people who don't move who are abnormal. They have given up their natural birthright—the right to move their own bodies.

It is now becoming increasingly obvious that we live in a culture that is somatically backwards and physically inhibited. In Asia, it is considered perfectly normal to move your body in public; the morning tai chi session in the park is routine and completely unremarkable. So forget the people around you; move like the animal you are.

In the end, it all comes down to a sense of priorities. What's more important to you, your cardiovascular system or the opinion of strangers? What's more important, the way you feel in your body or the way other people feel about your body? What's more important, taking advantage of a chance to play, or trying to look dignified in front of a sedentary public that has one foot in the grave? Yes, there are times for modesty and stealth, but if you won't move in public, you'll miss out on thousands of opportunities.

The corollary to this opportunistic philosophy comes from the Boy Scout motto: Be Prepared. We don't know when exercise opportunities will present themselves, so we had best be ready to grab them when we can. There are a number of simple strategies here: Wear multi-purpose clothing and shoes whenever possible so that if there's a chance to play, you'll be able to participate. Keep extra shoes in your car or under your desk. Keep a change of clothes and an extra towel in the trunk of your car so that you can clean up. Keep a Frisbee, a softball or a skateboard in your car.

Set up your office to take advantage of useless downtime. Get a headset for your telephone so you can stretch while they're keeping you on hold. Keep a dumbbell next to your desk; next time you're waiting for your computer to restart, you can squeeze off a couple of reps. Replace your office chair with a physioball; this will put some bounce into your normally static position and keep your spine happy.

finding time

When speaking of opportunity, we must also take a look at the world's most popular excuse for exercise avoidance; lack of time. Every trainer has heard this one thousands of times.

Granted, modern life puts excruciating demands on our schedules and most of us are pressed to the limit. But if we take a long view, we find that saving time by skipping exercise is just plain folly. If you think exercise takes too much time out of your life right now, consider the alternative. That is, try not moving for a few years and see how things balance out. In the short run, you'll be able to do all those other things that you absolutely must do and you'll be more productive. But in the long run, exercise avoidance will cost you more time than even the most intensive training program.

Sure, if you skip your movement session you'll be able to squeeze a few more hours out of your day and knock a few more things off your to-do list. But after a decade of being so productive, you'll find that you're spending a whole lot of time sitting in physician's waiting rooms and reading back issues of *People* magazine. You'll spend your mornings filling out insurance forms and waiting on hold, trying to get your provider to cover another round of physical therapy. You'll be limping the aisles at the local pharmacy, waiting to have another prescription filled. And instead of working and hanging out with your family and friends, you'll be down at the clinic, trying to get some function back into that ankle, knee, or hip. If you think that exercise is time-consuming, try injury! Sitting around with an ice-pack strapped to your body is not a good use of anyone's time.

And then there's the ultimate time waster, an early death. Sure, you can get a lot done if you just skip the movement classes and exercise sessions. You'll be really productive for a couple of decades or so. But then the grim reaper will come and take you away, years ahead of schedule. What a waste of time.

a little bit of something
is better than a whole lot of nothing

Here's another way to think about our perceived "time shortage." Working from the assumption that physical training takes a lot of time each week, a lot of people abandon the effort before their first workout. "Since I don't have 20 hours each week, I'm not going to get involved. It just takes too much time to get in shape." Sure, if you're trying to make the Olympic team, climb K2 or race in the Tour de France, you're going to need to put in thousands and thousands of hours. But what if you just want to be healthy and happy? Let's consider some modest, realistic efforts and multiply them out over the years and compare the result to a total non-effort.

Suppose that you run just 2 miles per week. This is a very modest program and it sure won't get you into competitive shape, but just look at these numbers: After one year you'll have run 104 miles. Keep at it and after ten years you will have logged 1040 miles. After 40 years, 4,160 miles. I don't have research results to confirm this, but my guess is that even this modest program is medically significant. I'd even bet that a physician would be able to measure the difference in your coronary arteries.

Or, suppose that you manage to hike 30 miles each summer, an easily achievable goal. After 40 years, that's 1,200 miles of hiking. Ride your bike just 10 miles each week; after 40 years that's 20,800 miles. Fifty push ups per week; that's 104,000 in 40 years. Stretch for thirty minutes each week: that's 1,040 hours of stretching in 40 years.

Granted, these modest efforts are not the ideal way to train for high performance; by spreading your efforts too thin, you won't stimulate major tissue changes and you certainly won't qualify for the Olympic team. Nevertheless, there will be an authentic physiological and psychological benefit. The occasional efforts will keep your muscle memory fresh. Compare the occasional athlete with the total slacker—there's a world of difference between "I haven't been running for 3 weeks" and "I haven't been running for 3 years." If it's been 3 weeks, you can reasonably expect to get back on track with minimal soreness. But if it's been 3 years, you might want to schedule an appointment with your physical therapist before you lace up your shoes.

All you can eat

We lived for days on nothing but food and water.

W.C. Fields

If you're anything like me, you're stuffed to the gills. You've been consuming in prodigious quantities and you should be satisfied, but you just can't stop. It feels like some vital tissue is about to rupture, but undaunted, you grab for one more bite.

What I'm talking about here is not food itself, but information about food. I'm talking about the books, the articles, the talk shows, the experts and the advice. I'm talking about the relentless rap that tells us that "Vitamin X is good for condition Y." I'm talking about the endless speculation about whether we need more or less protein, more or less red wine, more or less calcium. We can't go anywhere without having this fare heaped on our plates. The irony here is that, while we are stuffed with information about food, many of us don't really eat that well and many of us wind up feeling confused and guilty about the food we do eat.

If we listen to nutritional pundits, we are likely to come away with the idea that there is a single right way to eat and that they know what it is. We now have scores of books that tell us just how to do it: 40% of total calories from this substance, 30% from that substance, plus 500 milligrams of this other substance, and so on. These pundits would have us believe that they possess complete nutritional knowledge and that they know precisely what we ought to be eating.

Granted, we do have some solid working knowledge under our belts. We know how to prevent scurvy on long boat rides and, if we were to send our astronauts to the outer planets, we could probably supply them with a diet that would keep them going for a long time.

But even with our best science, we're a long, long way from nutritional certainty. Here's why:

First, people are different. We each have our own particular biochemistry and we each do different things with the foods that we eat. The variation can be huge. Some people can thrive on a low protein diet for example, but others will do poorly. And not only that, the way that we process food changes as we age. (As Heraclitus would have put it, "You can't put food into the same stomach twice.") What made you healthy when you were 10 might make you sick when you're 40.

Second, food also changes. Plants and animals change with the seasons and the locale. The beef that we eat today is not the same as the beef our parents ate and it is far higher in fat than the meat that our hominid ancestors ate. The vegetables that are grown in one region will have different micro-nutrients than those grown somewhere else.

Third we have the placebo effects. Most of us have heard about the placebo effect in a medical context, but placebo effects are at work throughout our lives and this is especially true in the world of food. If you believe that a particular food is good for you, it may actually give more nutritional value than something neutral. And of course, if you believe that a particular food is bad for you, it can have a nocebo effect and may actually prove detrimental. Food is not neutral; it has effects that reach far beyond the actual biochemical content. Complicating the matter even further is the fact that nutritional placebo effects are not constant throughout a person's life; they are always changing for each of us.

The fourth problem is that food is slow. Sure, we know the short-term effects of large doses of poisons, and the mid-term effects of protein malnutrition. But the things that concern many of us today—the nutritional factors involved in cancer and other degenerative diseases—take decades to manifest themselves. To put this in cybernetic terms, studying nutrition is like steering a large supertanker; actions don't show immediate results. You may change your diet for better or for worse, but you probably won't notice the effects for a long time.

And, to add yet one more layer to our already murky nutritional uncertainty, consider the fact that even the most sincere and honest nutritionists disagree on what's ideal. If specialists such as Robert Atkins and Dean Ornish can't come to agreement on the ideal human diet, then what are us nutritional mortals supposed to do?

For these reasons, no laboratory procedure or theoretical approach, no matter how sophisticated, can ever nail down the precise effects of the things that we eat. In this, there is simply no way we can make absolutist statements about food. All the books and experts who tell us that "substance X is good for condition Y" can never be more than partly right and often they'll be completely wrong.

the primal challenge

Lost in our hysteria over modern-day dieting, we have forgotten the fundamental issue. That is, the primal nutritional challenge, as experienced by most non-human animals and most humans throughout the vast reaches of biological history, is simply getting enough to eat. Obviously, environments vary over time; for any species, there will be periods of abundance and scarcity. But for most animals, the "problem of nutrition" is simply the problem of getting enough calories to stay alive. Famine is common in the animal world, and it has been common in human history as well. In this sense, if you're eating at all, you're eating well.

Blessed with fossil-fueled agriculture, we moderns are awash in things to eat. With the exception of certain localized regions, food is abundant; for many of us food is, for all practical purposes, free. But in our neurosis and paranoia, we have come to the conclusion that "good nutrition" consists of avoiding "bad" foods, especially "non-natural foods" that contain "toxins." This completely ignores the fact that, for the overwhelming majority of human history and for the rest of the natural world, "good nutrition" means "not starving to death." In this historical sense, all of our neurotic food combining, analyzing and supplementation completely misses the point.

This brings me to the Doug Scott diet. If you are familiar with the world of extreme mountaineering, you will recognize the name. Scott had a long and prolific career in the mountains, with many dramatic first ascents. When asked the key to his success, Scott replied that the reason he was able to thrive in such extreme environments was that he was able to eat pretty much anything that his mates brought along. ("Tuna fish and chocolate anyone?") In other words, he was a good omnivore and would have no doubt done well in a tribe of ancient hominids.

Now I say this somewhat in jest because, yes, there are undoubtedly some foods that we really ought to avoid–large quantities of saturated fat and insulin-busting carbohydrates are a good place to start. Nevertheless, the fact remains that today's nutritional focus is way off the mark. We are omnivores, and that as much as anything is the key to our evolutionary success. We are here today because, among other things, we can eat almost anything. If you look at the design of our digestive tract, you will see that the design is generalist: we can extract nutritional value from an astonishing range of substances. If you're an organism trying to survive in a hostile world of scarce resources, this is great news.

Nutritional fanatics like to promote idealized diets, of course, and they often resort to an automotive metaphor to explain their perspective. "Your body is like a high-performance race car; if you don't put high-quality fuel in the tank, you won't get the most out of it."

From an evolutionary perspective, this comparison completely misses the mark. The human body is actually more like a all-terrain Land Rover that can burn a multitude of fuels; diesel, gas, kerosene, maybe even vegetable oil. Sure, if you put the best fuels into it, it'll go a little faster and last a little longer, but ideal fuels aren't always available. If you're planning a trip across Africa, Asia and North American, you want a vehicle that can burn a multitude of fuels; you'd be crazy to take the Lamborghini.

William Leonard, professor of anthropology at Northwestern University has summed up the challenge of modern human nutrition this way:

> Too often modern health problems are portrayed
> as the result of eating "bad" foods that are de-
> partures from *the* natural human diet. This is
> a fundamentally flawed approach to assessing

human nutritional needs. Our species was not designed to subsist on a single, optimal diet...What is remarkable about human beings is the extraordinary variety of what we eat...The challenge our modern societies now face is balancing the calories we consume with the calories we burn. (*Scientific American* December, 2002)

the Pleistocene menu

So what did our primal ancestors eat? The short answer is to say "whatever they could." The long answer is more complex. To begin with, we know that most primates are vegetarian; we can assume that we share that metabolic heritage to some degree. Beyond that, consensus among paleoanthropologists is that our hominid ancestors did eat some meat on occasion and that this meat-eating probably spanned a range: the smaller, early hominids were largely vegetarian, but may have scavenged some meat. We surely ate whatever plants we could, depending on the locale and the season. It is a certainty that we ate roots, berries, fruits and nuts. Other primates eat these things routinely. Later, our larger, more contemporary ancestors may have eaten little else but meat.

Biological anthropologists tell us that three things were scarce in the hominid diet: fat, sugar and salt. This is not difficult to understand. Wild game meats are low in fat, considerably leaner than today's beef cattle; fat must have been a great delicacy.

There must have been some brief periods of abundant fresh, sugary fruits, and we can be sure that the hominid gang ate as much as they could. But such abundance would have been highly seasonal and certainly not part of the daily fare. In addition, there was no bread, no pasta, no jellies, cakes, cookies, cakes or soft-drinks. In other words, no high-octane foods that would cause radical insulin swings and metabolic flame-out.

The Paleolithic diet, if it was anything, was probably a slow-burn program with a low glycemic index; easy on the pancreas. A good Paleolithic feast, with fresh meat and local vegetables, would power the tribe for many hours at a stretch. Given the fact that this kind of diet worked for hundreds of thousands of years, it seems safe to assume that it would work for us moderns as well.

Unfortunately, we seem to be moving in the other direction. What we are seeing in today's modern diet is what has been called "cornification." Corn syrup, as you may know, is a sweet food additive. It is cheaper than sugar and has therefore become a popular ingredient in many food and food-like products. Some experts now estimate that corn syrup many constitute as much as 10% of the total calories consumed by modern Americans. Obviously, this is a huge departure from the primal diet, whatever it might have been. Given this dramatic increase in total calories derived from sugar and sugar-like substances, it comes as no surprise that we see an increase in adult-onset diabetes. We are building disease directly into our food supply.

the mosaic diet plan

Just as they do with exercise, some pundits advocate a data-intensive approach to nutrition. They tell us to start a food journal so that we can keep track of everything: calories, protein, fat, carbs, vitamins, minerals, fatty acids. In theory, if we could track every aspect of our nutritional lives, we could come up with an ideal diet. Of course, we'd be so busy entering numbers in our journals that we wouldn't have time to do much else. And even then, there would be no guarantee. Human nutritional physiology is intricately complex; like the earth's climate, it can vary wildly with even small changes in key variables.

A better course is to toss out the charts, the scale and the computer and imagine your ancestral life on the semi-wooded grassland. As we have speculated, the ancestral environment was probably a mosaic or patchwork of microhabitats, each with it's own particular set of edibles. On a day's journey, you would probably encounter several different kinds of food. Thus, the hominid diet probably varied considerably, not only with location, but also with the season. In other words, their diet was probably highly diverse.

Imagine your life in this mosaic habitat. Perhaps your tribe camped in a friendly valley for a few weeks. During that time you make short gathering trips each day and sampled the local fruits, vegetables and on occasion, animals. Maybe you ate a mono-diet for awhile, living on nothing but a certain orange-colored root. It was dull, but it kept you going. Later, the season changed and you moved to a new location where you found a new set of edibles that rounded out your diet and supplied what you'd been missing from your former menu. And, since hominids probably moved around a great deal, they must have eaten many different kinds of food. The mosaic environment gave them a diverse diet that probably supplied most of what they needed.

With this in mind, we might try structuring our diets in a similar fashion. Try creating your own miracle mosaic diet. Go to different "habitats," different neighborhoods, different restaurants. Eat around. Instead of popping vitamin pills to make up for possible deficiencies, eat new foods in new places. Even if you don't balance out every nutritional micro-ingredient, you'll at least enjoy the range of new tastes.

Try some mosaic-style shopping next time you go to the market. As you visit various section of the grocery store, imagine that the products come, not from different companies, but from different regions of your grassland habitat. Pick and choose as if you're on a walkabout. This mosaic program promises an easy, fun and tasty way to better nutrition. I have no research numbers to back up this claim, but my guess is that this kind of mosaic approach to eating is not only healthy, it is highly sustainable and pleasurable. In some regions, this kind of eating style is relatively easy. If you've got different neighborhoods in your city, you've got a mosaic of restaurants and cuisines to choose from.

The problem is that the trend in the modern food industry is in precisely the wrong direction, away from diversity and towards homogenization. Instead of maintaining locally diverse cuisine, fast food franchises now offer us precisely the same fare everywhere we go. We can now order exactly the same items in restaurants that are thousands of miles away from one another. This destroys the mosaic nutritional pattern that our bodies originally thrived upon.

This gives us yet another reason to avoid the fast food franchise. Not only do they serve up fare that is nutritionally questionable, they give us exactly the same stuff no matter whether we're in Seattle or Santa Fe. Not only do they serve up heaping plates of saturated fat and super-tanker cups of liquid carbohydrates, they simultaneously promote deficiencies and nutritional boredom by feeding us the same damn thing everywhere we go. Marketer researchers insist that consumers want a predictable dining experience, but maybe it's time we asked for some regional, mosaic diversity.

scarcity and abundance

For all animals, eating habits are linked to scarcity and abundance. In times of scarcity, the good animal eats what he can and is not particularly choosy. In times of plenty, he will eat more, but can also afford to be more discriminating. We know from observation that animals change their eating behavior to suit changing levels of scarcity and abundance. When times are hard, a grizzly bear will dig up roots out of the alpine meadow, but when there's elk around, he'll choose that instead.

Most modern humans live in a world of nutritional affluence. Since the advent of fossil-fuel powered agriculture, we have created a food environment of unprecedented abundance. Some of our food is low-quality to be sure and some of it is disease-promoting, but the fact remains that we are surrounded by calories.

The good animal response to hyper-abundance is to become more discriminating; if the bushes in the river valley are bent over and dripping with ripe fruit, it doesn't make sense to eat anything but the very finest. Unfortunately, many of us are poor animals in the midst of plenty. Instead of becoming more discriminating with the surplus, we continue eating nearly anything and make few choices on the basis of quality. This is our biggest nutritional mistake.

a matter of perspective

We can think of modern nutritional challenge as a "half full, half empty" situation. If you choose, you can look at today's nutritional environment and see food that is polluted with additives, antibiotics, refined carbohydrates and artery-clogging fats. You can see animal abuse, soil depletion and impending genetic catastrophe. Clearly, there is ample evidence of this point of view.

On the other hand, you can look our nutritional situation and see a cornucopia, an abundance of wonderful things to eat. This is also true. In comparison to many hominid populations, both historical and modern, we have a bountiful selection of extremely healthy foods all around us. If you're willing to be selective, you can find all sorts of foods that are bursting with flavor and physiological benefit. Never before in human history have so many people been able to eat so well.

It all depends on how you want to look at it. If you emphasize the negative, food becomes a nocebo, which further diminishes the value of what you're eating. If you look at the positive, food becomes a placebo and amplifies its already beneficial effects.

There's lots of evidence for both positions, of course, but personally, I prefer to see my plate as overflowing with wonderful, rich and nourishing foods. I am lucky. I can go to a local market and get tasty, nourishing food almost any time I want. Yes, there is a lot of seductive trash food out there, but all it takes is a little selectivity. You just have to be a little bit picky, that's all.

In any case, keep it simple. Seek balance by eating a diverse diet. Look for slow-burn foods that don't send you on wild insulin swings. Get some protein, some high-quality fats and as many fresh vegetables as you can. Last and most important perhaps, enjoy your food. If you've got abundance, celebrate. Tomorrow may be different.

Stress dance

It has now become a widely accepted belief that stress-reduction is a vital part of a complete health and fitness program. Today's health-conscious consumers understand that stress can have a negative effect on health and in turn, on fitness. Thus we seek out all sorts of stress-reducing disciplines, activities, substances and ideas. While this does seem to be a step in the right direction, it also obscures the fact that the relationship between stress, health and fitness is far more complex than most people think.

To understand how stress affects our bodies, we first need to take a quick look at the autonomic nervous system. This is the non-voluntary branch of the nervous system that regulates basic physiological functions such as breathing, cardiac output and digestion. There are two basic branches of the system: the sympathetic and the parasympathetic.

In the simplest terms, the sympathetic branch stimulates us for peak physical performance in time of crisis while the parasympathetic directs the rest and recovery process. All major organs are innervated by both kinds of fibers; it is the balance between them that determines our state of body and mind.

The sympathetic nervous system is famous for its "fight or flight" effect. When activated, it gives us that familiar rush of physical and mental energy, an exhilarating, even euphoric feeling. We experience an immediate arousal of the central nervous system which sets the stage for a host of other responses; muscle tone increases, respiration deepens and accelerates, heart rate increases and blood pressure rises. Blood is directed away from the digestive organs and toward the muscles where it is most urgently needed. The spleen dumps more red corpuscles into the bloodstream to carry additional oxygen and carbon dioxide. Fat and protein-rich tissues are broken down to create glucose. Chemicals are pumped into the blood to increase coagulation in anticipation of potential bleeding. Hormones are released to cause water retention by the kidneys in case of heavy sweating or blood loss. Taken together, there is no question that these sympathetic effects are desirable in physically demanding crisis situations. If you are a hunted-gatherer on the run, you want as much sympathetic activity as you can get.

This is no free physiological ride, however. The short term effects are clearly beneficial to a creature fighting for survival, but the long term effects may be something altogether different. When the body is under continuous, prolonged stress, the adrenal cortex begins to produce a hormone called cortisol. This hormone facilitates the adrenaline response so that body tissues become more sensitive to adrenaline's effects. This makes sense; the Paleolithic hunter who was chemically sensitized to adrenaline in a long-term physical challenge was more likely to survive.

So far, so good, but in the long term, the advantage fades away and can even reverse itself. High levels of cortisol dissolve collagen, the prime ingredient in connective tissues such as cartilage, tendons and ligaments. It also constricts blood vessels, reducing cellular oxygen supply. Tissues that are chronically oxygen deprived are forced to burn anaerobically, a process that generates lactic acid. This is slow to recycle and in the meantime, it festers, causing deep muscle soreness and possible tissue damage. And, to make matters worse, cortisol may also weaken the immune system, making us more susceptible to infection.

Cortisol also produces changes in metabolism. In sympathetic mode, the body stops digesting food and begins to use its own tissue for energy. Muscle and liver tissue are broken down to produce glucose; the body actually starts digesting itself. This is an efficient process and a good survival mechanism, but only up to a point; go too far and you will waste weeks or months of precious tissue development.

Modern discoveries in biochemistry suggest that accumulated long-term stress can be a serious threat to health and physical performance. Sustained production of cortisol interferes with the natural healing process, leads to adrenal exhaustion and drives a whole constellation of related health problems, especially the nasty over-use injury. In his book, *Job's Body*, Deane Juhan summed up the problem this way: "The very chemicals released by the body in order to safeguard itself in the case of emergency are the same ones whose long-term effects are demonstrably destructive, even fatal."

the virtues of fight and flight

Because of these recent discoveries in biochemistry, the "fight or flight" response has gotten a bad reputation in recent years and some people now go to great lengths to avoid stressful events of any kind. This is probably an over-reaction.

It's not the stress that's the problem, nor is it the stress response. Rather, it's the duration of the stress response and a lack of movement that eventually erodes tissue and health. Isolated stress events are easily tolerated by the body and may even be beneficial. Anecdotal evidence suggests that some measure of fight/flight experience may actually promote physical health. Stories from the mountain climbing community seem to bear this out. When climbers take on a large mountain, they fire their stress response repeatedly throughout the climb. Steep faces, exposed positions, hard climbing and loose rock are guaranteed to set off acute stress reactions as the body rallies to meet the challenge.

One might suppose that this stressful series of events would take a toll in the days to follow, but this is not necessarily what we see. In fact, many climbers report an enhanced state of health and vigor after a major climbing effort. Major physical stress, when experienced in the context of movement, appears to have therapeutic effects.

Paleolithic v. modern stress

At this point we are bound to wonder about the differences between Paleolithic and modern stress challenges. Obviously, this requires a fair amount of speculation and imagination, but we can make some realistic guesses.

On one level, life in the Paleolithic must have been blissfully simple and straightforward. No jobs, no money, no taxes. No noise, no traffic. No career to plan for, no retirement to save for. No college admissions, no layoffs. No telephone, no stock market. No waiting on hold, no computer crashes. In one sense, we can accurately describe the vast span of hominid experience as a 6 million year vacation.

Of course, our hominid ancestors also experienced some extremely urgent, non-negotiable physical challenges that could not be deferred, delayed or buffered by insurance. When the lion comes into camp in the middle of the night, you've got to move now. This kind of stress is acute.

For the modern human, the stress environment is entirely different: no predators, no wildfires, no competing with carnivores for freshly killed meat and, except in the case of the occasional natural disaster, no substantial exposure to heat or cold. Instead, we face an enormous, crushing burden of theoretical, abstract and conceptual stress. We get to worry about financial collapse, weapons of mass destruction, global warming, genetically modified foods, computer viruses, real viruses, corporate corruption, identity theft and stock options. These things aren't like lions. They don't strike in the night and leave in the morning; they linger, both in fact and in our imaginations. These stresses are best described as chronic.

In terms of stress and stress responses, the biggest difference between the Paleolithic and modern eras lies in the opportunity for movement. When the Paleolithic hunter-gatherer had a major stress event, his blood surged with high-octane hormones that mobilized him for action. But unless he got trapped in a tree or a cave, he'd probably have a ready opportunity to move and thereby flush any toxic chemicals out of his system. "You should have seen it! A leopard almost got me today! I was so freaked that I was shaking. My heart was blasting, my palms were cold and sweaty and my mind was racing. But after I escaped, I ran all the way back to camp and by the time I got there, I felt a lot better."

In contrast, we have the perpetually panicked modern. "I scrambled to send in my quarterly tax statement, but the deadline was coming up and it looked like I was going to get audited. I tried to email it in, but I forgot my password and then my computer crashed. I finally got the whole thing sorted out, but the traffic on the way home was gridlocked and now I've got to get that report ready for tomorrow, and no, I don't have time to go for a walk!" The difference: The Paleolithic hunter gets to flush his bloodstream, the worried modern gets to stew.

Technically, the hunted-gatherer's encounter with the predator was more physically stressful, but because he has fewer opportunities for movement, the stresses experienced by the modern human are probably more corrosive. The message? Get some exercise, especially when the world is closing in on you.

ignore false triggers

It's not that we need to eliminate the sympathetic response. Rather, we need to synchronize the activity of the autonomic system with the activities that we're involved in. The idea is to get the right autonomic response at the right time; sympathetic when we need physical powers, parasympathetic when we're relaxing. What we are after is a sense of physiological control, balance and regulation.

The problem is that the sympathetic system is highly sensitive and easily activated; it's a self-amplifying, positive feedback system. When stimulated by real or perceived danger, the adrenal cortex produces adrenaline, which, in addition to acting on the target organs, acts as a neurotransmitter which provides more stimulation to the sympathetic system as a whole. This in turn stimulates the production of more adrenaline and so on. Activation of the sympathetic response is easy, which from an evolutionary standpoint, is as it should be. When a carnivore is chasing you through the bush, you need all the sympathetic amplification you can get. Thus, it only takes a small nudge to set the process in motion and once moving, it goes fast.

The problem with this hair-trigger sensitivity is that not only will the body fire a sympathetic response to an actual physical crisis, it will also fire it when challenged by perceived threats, even ones that are entirely non-physical, even ones that have no relevance to your survival. Thus, just about anything can set it off; a sharp word from a spouse or co-worker, a conflicting idea in the newspaper, a belligerent voice on talk radio and most famously, the erratic driving behavior of people on the road. From the body's point of view, all of these are treated as predator attacks.

In the modern world, the thing we want to avoid is setting off the sympathetic system unnecessarily. To some extent, we can do this simply by recognizing false alarms for what they are. Next time you face a challenge, ask yourself "Is this an authentic threat to my body? Is this a valid trigger?" That aggravating voice on talk radio is certainly annoying, but it is not a predator. That looming deadline at work will definitely challenge your ability to organize your time, but it is not a wildfire. There is no physical threat to your body in these cases and little will be gained by firing your sympathetic system. Let it go. Save your stress response for when you really need it.

When you start looking around, you'll find that there are thousands of false triggers out there that you can safely ignore. As soon as you recognize false triggers as such, you'll gain a new measure of control over your physiology and your health.

feed and breed, tend and befriend

In describing the flip side of the flight/fight response, some people have take to describing the parasympathetic response as "feed and breed" or "tend and befriend." This description acknowledges the comforting effects of social support and companionship. Relaxing with the tribe is a place of refuge and safety. As you enter this refuge, your sense of urgency fades and your body relaxes. The predatory threats to your well-being have been dealt with for the time being and now you can pamper your body.

In contrast to the hair-trigger setting of the sympathetic system, the parasympathetic nervous system is less easily activated. There is less survival urgency here and consequently, it's not nearly so sensitive. From an evolutionary standpoint, this makes sense. When you're on the grassland, there's no pressing, urgent need to relax.

Consequently, some of us have difficulty transitioning out of fight-flight into feed-breed; we tend to get stuck in the sympathetic mode. Fortunately, there are several simple strategies we can use to promote relaxation.

Breathing is good place to begin. Breathing creates a distinct physiological response that moderates the sympathetic response. Every full movement of the diaphragm massages the internal organs and promotes circulation. This is a lesson that is easily forgotten in times of stress, but it does produce results.

Pampering is essential to parasympathetic rejuvenation. To repair itself, the animal body wants to feel safe, secure and content.To support this cycle we can turn to the time-honored methods of meditation, massage, exercise and social support. These are essential nurturing arts. Find one that works for you and practice it.

Activate the parasympathetic with intentional, conscious rest and rejuvenation. Get yourself into a quiet place with good friends, good food and spare time. Activate the "feed and breed" response and let your body heal itself. This will not win you any glamour or achievement awards, but it will keep you in the game a lot longer - it could even save your life.

Keeping a balanced perspective

Not only do we seek a physical sense of equilibrium, we also look to balance the overall perspective that we bring to our physical training and experience. We want the agility and grace to move smoothly through the world, but we also want to maintain a balanced attitude about what we're doing.

One particularly valuable way to approach this is to look at Robert Pirsig's romantic and classical points of view. In *Zen and the Art of Motorcycle Maintenance*, Pirsig took us on a philosophical cross-country journey which featured a deep reflection on these two perspectives. Pirsig didn't say much about health or fitness, but his discussion fits our purposes perfectly. For Pirsig, the distinction breaks down this way:

> A classical understanding sees the world primarily as underlying form itself. A romantic understanding sees it primarily in terms of immediate appearance...The romantic mode is primarily inspirational, imaginative, creative, intuitive. Feelings rather than facts predominate...The classic mode, by contrast, proceeds by reason and by laws–which are themselves underlying forms of thought and behavior...

We recognize the classic perspective when we hear people speak about systems, schematics, flow charts, hierarchies, sequences, units, precision and quantity. Stereotypically, we think of engineers, although engineers can have their romantic side too. In contrast, we recognize the romantic perspective as one that emphasizes appearance, experience, aesthetics, passion, wildness, sensation and quality. Stereotypically, we think of artists, although artists can have their classic side as well.

For the fitness enthusiast, it's easy to see these qualities in the way people approach exercise and conditioning. On one hand we have the romantic. Here we imagine the dancer, an individual who is primarily interested in the quality of his or her movement. He speaks the language of passion, feeling, expression and inspiration. When the romantic exerciser steps into the gym, the studio or onto the stage, he is looking to create an experience with meaning. For him, quality movement is considered an end in itself. If it feels good, it probably is good.

On the other hand we have the exercise physiologist and the fitness scientist. These individuals focus their attention on data, quantification and measurable results. When the classical exerciser steps into the gym, the studio or onto the practice field, he looks to achieve a certain performance result. The immediate experience is less important than the ultimate outcome. For him, practice sessions are considered to be a means to an end, typically a record-setting performance or a trip to the Finals.

It's easy to see that individual exercisers have distinct preferences for classic or romantic points of view. In the extreme, it works like this: The romantic prefers dance, yoga, aikido and tai chi and wouldn't be caught dead with a clipboard. He consistently looks for the experiential quality of movement and has no interest in keeping score or breaking records.

The classicist, on the other hand, tends to prefer weight lifting, running, swimming or any other activity that can be readily quantified, broken down, analyzed, tabulated and cross-referenced. He derives a sense of satisfaction from recording his performance and comparing it to previous efforts. For the classical extremist, the numbers may even become more important than the experience itself.

Naturally, each of these schools of thought tend to have a negative opinion of the other. Classicists consider the romantics to be empty-headed dabblers who prefer abstraction and mysticism to authentically challenging movement. They see the romantic style as nothing more than a lofty-sounding dodge, something people do to avoid the genuine work that is necessary for physical improvement.

Romantics, on the other hand, view the classicists as insensitive automatons who bear a strong resemblance to the machines they work with such devoted labor. They may have the right numbers, but if you take their clipboards away, they have nothing left. Pirsig described the conflict this way:

> To a romantic, this classic mode often appears dull, awkward and ugly. Everything's got to be measured and proved. Oppressive. Heavy. Endlessly grey. The death force. Within the classic mode, however, the romantic has some appearances of his own. Frivolous, irrational, erratic, untrustworthy, interested primarily in pleasure seeking. Shallow. Of no substance.

And, when it gets really nasty, it breaks down this way: the romantic attempts to claim the mysto-spiritual high ground, usually talking about the power of intuition to trump the wicked and soulless machinery of the classicist. The classicist, for his part, lays claim to scientific certainty, backing it up with reams of data, footnotes and references. It's worth noting that in the fitness marketplace, both of these extremes seem to flourish. Fitness consumers seem attracted to both poles for their own reasons, while the middle ground looks pretty thin.

It's easy to get wrapped up in this debate between competing perspectives, but a couple of points stand out. First, if you're really serious about creating a life of sustainable health and fitness, both the romantic and classical perspectives are necessary and neither one is sufficient. Either one, if pursued exclusively, will lead to boredom, performance plateaus and probable injury. Each extreme leads to absurdity.

On one hand, if we do nothing but concentrate on creating a spiritually-based, intuitive movement experience, we'll eventually get lost in the stratosphere of abstraction and our performance will drift aimlessly. The body, especially the nervous system, needs a fairly regular cycle of challenge, repetition and rest to make tissue changes. If we simply do what feels right, we probably won't get very far. On the other hand, if we do nothing but log thousands of miles, sets and reps, we will eventually die of boredom (and bore our friends to death as well).

Truly experienced coaches recognize the fact that we need to oscillate between the romantic and classical poles. Phil Jackson, coach of the champion Chicago Bulls and Los Angeles Lakers, is a prime example. Jackson has long been celebrated in the sports media as the "Zen Master," a coach who constantly urges his players to seek the mystical and spiritual qualities of the basketball experience. But don't be deceived. Jackson works his players hard, and you can bet that someone in his organization is carrying a clipboard, dutifully counting training details. You don't get a handful of championship rings on a diet of mysticism alone.

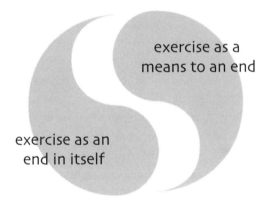

So, with balance in mind, what we're looking for is a way to bring both of these perspectives together into a single method that honors the entire spectrum of possibility. Yes, we need to talk about passion, sensation and quality of movement, but we're also have to talk about sets, reps and exercise science. We're need to work, but we're need to play too.

Draw on both sources. If you're a dedicated clipboard jockey, you might want to spend a little more time on the romantic side of physical training. Go for the sensation, not the numbers. Tend to the experience first. Think process before achievement. Write a poem about your sport, sing about your training. Create new games and variations. You just might find a renewed sense of interest in what you're doing.

If you're a romantic athlete, you may want to balance out your efforts with some sustained, disciplined physical striving; ie, work. Forget the experience for awhile; go out and get some good numbers. Write down your stats. Make a spreadsheet and fill in the little boxes with sets and reps; you'll be amazed how hard some of the classical athletes are working.

Exercising freedom and discipline

One of the longest-running debates in the education and fitness community hinges on the relative importance of freedom and discipline. Discipline advocates believe that the human body, if left to it's own instincts, will either languish on a performance plateau or degenerate into sloth and weakness. Therefore, they put their trust in methodology, form, sets and reps. Stick to the program and you'll get results.

Freedom advocates on the other hand, believe that the body knows best and that physical intuition is a reliable and dependable teacher. As long as you're participating, you'll be making progress. Just do what comes naturally and you'll be doing it right. Naturally, these two camps come into frequent conflict.

Enter Alfred North Whitehead. Whitehead was a British philosopher (1861-1947), who wrote some practical and sensible material on education. His primary interest was academic, scholastic education, but as you will see, his observations apply equally to education of all varieties, physical education included. One gem really stands out, his essay "The Rhythmic Claims of Freedom and Discipline."

Whitehead saw a fundamental duality between freedom and discipline in the educational process. In his view, each quality is considered essential. "The only avenue towards wisdom is by freedom in the presence of knowledge. But the only avenue towards knowledge is by discipline in the acquirement of ordered fact." In other words, you've got to cut people loose to explore, but you've also got to narrow their focus and keep them on track. Every teacher lives and dies by balancing these competing needs.

To reconcile the contradictory values of freedom and discipline, Whitehead urged a dynamic oscillation, a rhythm between the two that allows both to flourish. "The two principles, freedom and discipline, are not antagonists, but should be so adjusted in the child's life that they correspond to a natural sway, to and fro, of the developing personality...all mental development is composed of such cycles, and of cycles of such cycles." The method is always in motion.

For Whitehead, the first phase of the cycle is what he called the "Stage of Romance." Here the student is given the freedom to explore and develop a sense of interest. The teacher is there, not to "teach" or lecture as we generally think of it, but only to stoke the fire. Here, curiosity is the prime mover. Success is achieved when students find passion in the material and the process. This is a time of play and exploration, not of tests or grades.

The second part of the cycle is the "Precision Stage." This is the time for narrowing the field of attention and tightening the focus. This is the time for right answers and sound logic. This is also the time for grades, exams and evaluations. This stage is dominated by discipline and rigor. It may not be fun, but it is essential.

The final period is what Whitehead calls the "Stage of Generalization." This is closely related to romance phase, except that now the field is seen by the student with a new set of facts or tools. Here the process returns to passion, curiosity and interest, but with the ability to go deeper than before.

According to Whitehead, every educational experience, from the child's piano lesson to the rigors of a graduate degree, ought to follow this rhythmic sway. Unfortunately, much of this rhythm, if it ever existed, has been ground up in the gears of standardization, and now every classroom and gymnasium looks pretty much the same from minute to minute and month to month. Instead of a rhythmic sway, we have a monotonous constancy.

Whitehead's primary concern was with academic education, but we can be sure that he would have had similar observations about physical education. When we apply Whitehead's principles to our physical training, we move from cycle to cycle, alternating between freedom and discipline. The warm-up thus becomes a time of spontaneity, of play, freedom and even, as Whitehead describes it, romance. The message here is simple. Start your session with freedom and liberation; move the way you want to move. In this, there is no right way to warm up. Explore the directions, speeds, sensations and intensities that make sense to you. In other words, play. There is no scientifically correct method here; only the method that captures your own bodily interest.

Eventually, of course, you'll have to tighten up your act. After fifteen minutes of productive messing around, it's time to get into the precision stage. During this phase, you'll take a small set of movements and hone them to the greatest possible perfection. It doesn't matter what particular quality you're after here—speed, strength, agility or endurance—this is the time for maximum concentrated effort. As Whitehead put it, "The stage is dominated by the inescapable fact that there are right ways and wrong ways, and definite truths to be known." Here the instructor must tighten the screws and set exacting standards. This is the "just so" phase of training. It is demanding and difficult. This is the time for the coach to apply pressure and demand excellence.

Later in the session, the need for discipline fades away, the nervous system fatigues and the process returns to play. Ideally, you'll be able to apply the new movement skills right away, but even if you can't, you'll still finish the session with a sense of interest and freedom that should carry you over to the next work-out. The cycling is crucial to advancement and motivation. "The organism will not absorb the fruits of the task unless its powers of apprehension are kept fresh by romance."

We can apply Whitehead's oscillation to any time scale we wish. It makes good sense to pattern the individual workout as romance-precision-romance or play–precision–play. You can also set up a sporting season in a similar fashion—a pre-season of movement exploration and casual fun, followed by a period of intensive rigor, followed by the playoffs—a time to unite the best of both into precision play. And, you may even want to structure your entire career this way, moving from a playful youth to precision adulthood, followed by a playful maturation.

Be a good animal

Vertebrate, mammal, primate, hominid, *Homo sapiens*. Like it or not, we are animals. We are unique to be sure, but so is every other species. We have unique bodies and special abilities, but so do dolphins, bats and leopards.

We can learn all the exercise science we want. We can learn all the details of glucose tolerance, metabolic pathways, oxygen uptake and amino acid balance. We can buy all the latest graphite, titanium toys and hire a squad of personal trainers and coaches, but unless we honor our animal nature, we'll never achieve the kind of fitness and primal vitality that we're capable of. We are animals and it's about time we got good at it.

two valued thinking

Unfortunately, the human mind is notorious for falling into the trap of either-or, two-valued thinking. We say that things must be either one way or the other way; black or white, A or not-A. In following this reasoning, we have managed to convince ourselves that humans and non-human animals inhabit two distinct and mutually exclusive classes. You're a member of either one class or the other; you're either a human or an animal. This pigeon-holing of humans and animals has been particularly popular over the last 400 years or so.

And so, when we say the word "animal," we tend to think "other" or even "alien." Given as we are to black and white, xenophobic thinking, we cast the situation in polarized opposites. There's "us" and "them." And some of us go even further, concluding that since we are intelligent, they must be stupid and since we are valuable, they must be worthless.

But this is a false and dangerous dichotomy that warps our behavior and stunts our intelligence. In our two-valued logic, we assume that if we become less animal-like, we simultaneously become more human. And by the same token, we assume that if we were to somehow become more animal-like, we would simultaneously become less human.

But this is an error of faulty categorization. It is not only possible to be fully animal and fully human simultaneously; it is desirable. What we need is a unification of human and animal qualities. In this, a good human is a good animal. Becoming more animal-like is perfectly consistent with human development.

be a good animal

So we're wondering what it means to "be a good animal." This can get confusing, especially if we consult the biologists. They'll give us a Darwinian explanation and offer up the idea that a "good animal" is one that produces a large number of viable offspring, thereby transporting his or her genes into the future. This explanation, while biologically correct, is not exactly what we're looking for here. What we're looking for is an orientation to our bodies and a relationship to the world that keeps us vigorous, vibrant and physically happy.

Being a good animal is mostly a matter of getting your priorities straight. It means, among other things, placing high value on the state of your body. It means giving your body what it needs and what it wants. Non-human animals are masters of this art. The good animal is assertive in getting what it needs, whether it be the right food, the right companionship or the right amount of movement. Obviously, we can't always get all of what we want, but we can usually get some of what we need. Being a good animal means making the effort.

biophilia

Above all, the good animal is a biophiliac. As described by biologist E. O. Wilson, biophilia (literally "love of life") is our "innate tendency to affiliate with other living creatures and processes." The natural world keeps us healthy and in turn, probably promotes physical performance as well. Hospital studies show that patients with a window view of trees in a natural setting had shorter post-operative stays, fewer complications and requested less pain medication than those who had a view of a brick wall. And we have all heard about the beneficial effects of pets on sick human patients. It is obvious that contact with trees, dirt, rocks and animals is good for us.

Evidence for biophilia as a genuine human attribute is now beginning to come to light. In *The Biophilia Hypothesis*, Roger Ulrich reviewed studies of human landscape preference. He found that "observers prefer forest settings having some similarities to savanna-like or parklike settings, including visual openness and uniform ground cover associated with large-diameter mature trees and relatively small amounts of slash and downed wood." Whether we're conscious of it or not, we seem to prefer landscapes that offer easy bipedal living. It hardly seems like a coincidence that we spend millions of dollars and hours of labor caring for lawns in front of our homes; we're keeping a piece of the Serengeti with us wherever we go.

Ulrich also cites studies analyzing the effects of outdoor scenes on stressed individuals. His findings suggest that "viewing un-threatening landscapes tends to produce faster and more complete restoration from stress than does viewing unblighted urban or built environments lacking nature." Apparently, natural settings tend to stimulate the parasympathetic nervous system, that branch of the nervous system associated with rejuvenation and tissue repair. One hospital study found that patients exposed to "serene" landscape pictures showed significant reductions in blood pressure. Another study of suggested that patients responded more positively to wall art dominated by natural content, but tended to react negatively to abstract painting and prints. A prison study found that inmates with a view towards nearby farms and forests were less likely to report for sick call than those whose cell windows faced the prison yard.

These results point us towards the inescapable conclusion that, in some subtle way, nature is medicine. It also suggests that, if natural settings are good for your health, they're likely to be good for your fitness as well. Of course, we could also see it from the other side. That is, it's not so much that natural landscapes have a positive effect on the human mind and body. Rather, it's that non-natural land-scapes have a negative effect. Our current state of ill health is at least partly the result of being forced to live in environments that have no resemblance to our natural habitat.

When we hear talk about biophilia, some of us are inclined to take the root words—love and life—and get carried away. Today's urbanites are so remote from the natural world that they can get away with projecting whatever qualities they want onto nature. Thus we romanticize nature, imagining it as some perfect, beneficent utopia where everything is in balance. We see glorious nature photos in glossy magazines and think of the natural world as a uniformly peaceful, soothing and stress-free place, full of colorful plants and wise and moral animals.

In fact, anyone who has had a sustained encounter with the natural world will tell an entirely different story. Nature, as it turns out, is not some nurturing being that will cradle us in it's arms and hold us until we feel better. No, nature is what it wants to be; sometimes friendly, sometimes indifferent, sometimes outrageously hostile and horrifying. Many times, it seems that nature is simply trying to do its level best to kill us.

When E.O. Wilson talks about biophilia, he is not talking about a squishy, romantic love of pretty sunsets. Rather, he is talking about a deep physical, primal need for contact. The word he uses repeatedly is *affiliation.* Just as social animals have a strong need to maintain contact with their fellows, so too do we have a drive to touch our living environment. Romance has nothing to do with it. What our bodies want is contact with plants, animals, rolling terrain and open sky. Our senses crave this stuff. We need to smell the land, touch the dirt with our bare feet, feel the textures of the plants, see the movement of the animals, and feel the wind on our faces.

Paradoxically, nature seems to be a healing force even when it presents us with difficult, challenging and life-threatening conditions. Encounters with the natural world appear to be generally therapeutic, even when they are unpleasant. (Some might even say *especially* when they are unpleasant.) The biophiliac's main interest is in developing and maintaining contact and affiliation with the living world of plants, animals, land and sky; this contact does not need to be pleasant to be valuable.

Massage therapists frequently speak of the power of touch in human health. We know, for example, that infants who are touched frequently grow larger and healthier, while infants who are touch-deprived fail to develop normally. As social animals, we thrive on physical human contact, but there seems to be an even wider need that goes beyond our species. We need to touch, smell and see living things of all varieties; in a sense, we need to be massaged by the natural world. We need to be massaged by driving rain, blinding sun, steep terrain and long distances. When we are deprived of this contact, our health suffers.

born to be wild

Back in the Pleistocene, all hominids–including humans–were wild animals. In fact, we have been wild animals for the vast majority of our history–intelligent, wild, bipedal animals.

Life on the grassland was wide open. We could go where we wanted and behave according to our desires. There were no laws, no rules, no borders, no regulations. Tribal living did limit our behaviors in some ways, of course. The elders surely exercised their authority and our peers must have applied their pressures, but in general we were highly independent creatures. We were physical, active and alert. We formed our own opinions, asked our own questions and made up our own minds about what we wanted to do. We were not easily herded, led or managed. Tribes must have broken up and reformed repeatedly on the grassland. We were natural anarchists.

Our wildness began to fade with the rise of agriculture; the invention of the hoe changed everything. As we began to work the soil, we spent more time in single locations. No longer free to roam in search of food, we tethered ourselves to the fields and the villages that grew up around them. Not only did we begin to domesticate certain non-human animals, we also began to domesticate ourselves.

There were obvious benefits to this self-imposed domestication, but the cost was high. We gained a reliable food supply, literacy, art, mathematics, science and high culture, but we gave up a significant measure of our animal independence. After several centuries of accepting this bargain, we have become pliable and leadable, not unlike the domesticated creatures that we keep in our fields and stockyards.

Giving up our wildness has given us great comforts, knowledge and amusements, but it has been disastrous for our bodies. As we allow ourselves to channeled and herded from one sedentary activity to another, we give up the movement that keeps us alive. Herded by the ever more insidious influences of marketing and advertising, we now drift from sedentary jobs to sedentary entertainment, then back again.

At one point in history, we could have made a good case for some degree of self-domestication. Sacrificing some of our liberty paid off handsomely in industrial efficiency, material rewards and physical comfort. But as usual, the dose makes the poison. At some point, the willingness to go with the herd becomes positively pathological to our minds and our bodies. By giving up our wildness, we also give up a powerful source of physical and creative inspiration. This, as much as anything else, has led to our poor physical condition.

the domestication of exercise

We can see our domestication clearly in the modern exercise world. State-of-the-art air-conditioned facilities with perfect ergonomics, juice bar and drop-in classes are designed to make fitness as easy as possible. There is no authentic challenge involved here, no inconvenience, no risk and ultimately, no satisfaction. Participants know in advance exactly what they are going to be doing in a training session and the surprises are few. These programs have been stripped of physical risk and psychological uncertainty. They adhere to regular schedules and follow set routines of choreographed movements. Domesticated clinics and gym environments provide a comfortable setting for health maintenance and socializing, but nothing more. Boredom is high and so is attrition. But since there's no challenge, there can be no enduring satisfaction. No satisfaction, no reason to come back.

This explains the recent trend in fitness, the increasing popularity of extreme, high-risk sports such as rockclimbing, whitewater kyaking and alpine snowboarding. While these activities are fairly absurd pursuits in their own right, they do have an appeal that you'll never find in a chrome-plated gym; that is, the outcome is not guaranteed.

The same holds true for the continuing appeal of martial art and the new fitness boot camps. Combative practice is inherently risky; you never really know what your opponent will do. Nor, in many cases, do you know what your instructor will demand. Thus, students experience a sense of wildness and unpredictability. Success, when it comes, tends to be extremely satisfying and participation tends to stick.

domestication by television

In the old days, we used to domesticate one another by sheer force; do what you're told or get whacked. Today we control one another by more subtle means, especially with colorful patterns of light that flicker across our TV screens, attracting our attention as lures attract fish.

As a culture, we are massively entertained, living on a steady diet of TV, movies and videos. Americans spend millions of hours watching TV each year. If nothing else, these hours of inactivity go a long way towards our state of atrophy. If you're living on the couch, you're not going to be burning calories or stimulating your physiology.

But the sheer number of hours spent in front of the screen may actually be a minor part of television's ill effect on our bodies. Yes, if you lay on the couch for hundreds of hours each year, it is inevitable that your physical condition will deteriorate. But those hours of viewing aren't just neutral entertainment; they also include a vast number of carefully-crafted images that tell us how to think about our bodies. They suggest that the world is populated by perfectly sculpted supermodels and athletes and that the path to health is through products, supplements and pharmaceuticals.

This creates a profound sense of unease, anxiety and frustration. Convinced that we can never measure up to the rarefied images we see before us, many of us simply give up on our bodies and live vicariously through the images of beauty and athletic achievement that are pumped into our homes. The dissonance between the idealized images before us and the actual characteristics of normal human bodies tweaks our brains. Kalle Lasn, author of *Culture Jam* and founder of *Adbusters* suggests that, "chronic TV watching is North America's number one mental health problem." As it turns out, it may also be our at the root of our physical condition as well.

reclaiming our wildness

If we're going to reclaim our health we are going to have to reclaim some of our wildness. This means reasserting our independence, thinking for ourselves, questioning authority and asking difficult questions. It means rebelling against domestication.

This is not to suggest that we ought to cut all ties to the modern world and go feral. I am not suggesting that we should strip off our clothes and wander the landscape in search of food, mates and excitement. Some degree of restraint is required.

What we can do is strive for a hybrid approach, the civilized-wild man advocated by Thoreau. In this, we would combine the primal animal with the civilized and cultured sophisticate. The ideal man, he believed, drew on both the wild and the refined. He strove to make himself "half-cultivated." "I would not have every part of a man cultivated, any more than I would have every acre of earth." Thus he sought to live "a sort of border life," a liminal life.

The idea here is to keep one foot planted firmly in the Pleistocene, the other planted in the heart of civilized culture. Become bilingual. Speak the language of the body and become fluent in vigorous movement. Then speak the language of the sophisticated; art, music science.

Keep the contrast clear. A civilized philosophy implies the pursuit of such ideas as truth, justice and beauty. It suggests the ability to understand and converse in commonly accepted conventions and the willingness to engage in fair and rational discourse. It implies the willingness to adjust behaviors towards peaceful co-existence as well as living with decency, fairness, sincerity, compassion

In contrast, domestication suggests a habitual pattern of followership, indoor living and passivity. It includes a compulsive obedience to authority, convention and tradition; a reflexive herding behavior. Domestication often includes a long-term commitment to 24-hour, year-round, indoor living. It also implies an internalization of the social taboo against public physical movement and pleasure. These qualities are not only bad for your health, they also happen to be bad for social living and cultural progress. While we can never be too civilized, it is easy to be too domesticated.

exercise deviance

In today's world, the biggest challenge in trying to be physically fit is that our entire technological and cultural infrastructure is set up specifically to provide us with the exact opposite of what we need to succeed. Our tools and machines are intentionally designed to relieve us of the physical movement and kinetic stresses that keep us healthy. Not only that, these tools and machines have been integrated into our culture to such an extent that their use is basically unavoidable. As the Surgeon General's report stated:

> The major barrier to physical activity is the age in which we live. In the past, most activities of daily living involved significant expenditures of energy. In contrast, the overarching goal of modern technology has been to reduce this expenditure through the production of devices and services explicitly designed to obviate physical labor.

This means that fitness is now a problem much deeper than sets, reps and tips. Rather, it's a problem of how we choose to live in modern culture. This in turn demands that we take on issues of conformity, obedience, independence and ultimately, wildness. If we're going to be fit or healthy in this modern age, we're going to have to be subversive, deviant or eccentric to some degree.

This makes the fitness challenge doubly difficult. Not only do we have to learn the fundamentals of movement and find the time to practice them, we also have to buck the cultural and technological infrastructure that keeps us pinned to our chairs and trapped in our automobiles. In this sense, fitness is not a mainstream activity; it is profoundly counter-cultural.

When our world becomes fully automated and sedentary living becomes the norm, deviance becomes a prerequisite for health. If you want to be vigorous and physically fit, you're going to have to behave differently from the people around you. If you're not willing to be at least slightly deviant from the culture at large, your fitness and your health are going to suffer.

Our situation stands in extreme contrast to the social and cultural conditions experienced by hunting, fishing and gathering humans in the Pleistocene. For these people, tribal culture gave total support physical movement and thus, good health. No deviance was necessary because movement was woven into everyday life. People encouraged one another to move, hunt, play and dance. We were rewarded for movement.

But when our cultural and technological infrastructure is set up to relieve us of physical labor and thus eliminate our fitness, it becomes clear that deviance is essential for health, just as necessary as food and water. In this sense, fitness is not a mainstream activity. Rather, taking care of yourself is a radical act.

Conventional fitness publications often describe some variation of the "three pillars of fitness," often listing them as aerobic capacity, strength and flexibility. But given the context and the environment in which we live, we would do just as well to say that the three pillars of fitness are "mischief, deviance and rebellion."

When you take this approach to health and fitness, you may find yourself losing interest in things like exercise spreadsheets, sets, reps and schedules. You'll get tired of fitness authorities who tell you about "proper form." Tigers and wolves don't need instruction in movement, why should you? Fitness is something that you already know how to do.

In this way, every movement session takes on a deeper meaning. When you go for a run, you're not just burning calories, you're creating culture. Every workout becomes both an act of affirmation and an act of defiance. Every play session an expression of joy and rebellion. By moving vigorously and frequently, you become an activist, not only for your own personal health and happiness, but for social progress.

Every time you do a movement session, you defy the forces that would have us become disembodied, robotic consumers. Every time you turn off the TV, you silence the voices of domestication that will sap your strength. Every time you play, you laugh at the tyrants of labor who would have us work around the clock until we die.

Now maybe you relish the idea of being a subversive or a deviant. If so, you're off to a good start. You'll have no problem walking when you could be riding, taking the stairs when everyone else is riding the elevator or doing stretching exercises while you're waiting for the bus. But if you're not comfortable with social deviance, you may need some practice. Regular movement is a good place to start. Try stretching in public. Do calisthenics in the parking lot. Skip the movie and go for a walk.

expose yourself

The antidote to domestication is exposure. In other words, get out. Break out of your house, get out of the car and out of the gym. Do your living and your playing outdoors whenever possible. Get wet, dirty, hungry and thirsty. Fill your lungs with fresh air. Hiking is the ultimate biophilic exercise program. One hour of hiking on a rocky trail is worth ten hours on the treadmill. One hour of swimming in a cold mountain lake is worth a hundred hours in a chlorine-saturated pool. One hour standing in front of a campfire is worth a million hours of television.

Do whatever it takes to make this happen for yourself. Buy the best outdoor clothing you can afford. Spare no expense on tents and sleeping bags. Get the best footwear you can and learn how to take care of your feet. Fight the traffic to get out of town or schedule your life to get out at the off-peak times.

Feed your appetite for exploration. Imagine yourself living in the ancestral landscape, the mosaic environment of human origins. Each valley held new plants, animals and a baffling variety of hominids. Curiosity would have driven you across the grassland and over the distant ridge just as surely as predators or bad weather. As the forests thinned out and the grassland came into view for the first time, our primate ancestors must have looked out in wonder. The horizon began to unfold, and we beheld the wider world for the first time. What is out there?

As bipedalism gave us the means, we began to explore the mosaic habitat before us. The more we explored, the more curious we became. New terrain, new plants and animals. New tribes of hominids with strange appearances and behaviors. So compelling was our curiosity that we eventually left the grassland in waves of migration and went in search of more novelty, making the journey from Olduvai to Europe, Asia and North America in a mere few thousand years.

do something unnatural

Living in an alien environment as we do, we find ourselves in a predicament. Given the fact that we are essentially hard-wired to prefer rest and idleness to sustained movement and that our modern world is set up to give us exactly what we want, it starts to become obvious that if we want to stay healthy through movement, we're going to have to do something that in a sense, feels wrong. We're going to have to go against our wiring.

Some people get around our out-of-context conundrum by dedicating themselves to absurdist pursuits such as mountain climbing, long-distance running and cross-continental backpack trips. Obviously, these pursuits are non-essential to survival in the modern world; no one need to climb a mountain, row across the ocean or ride their mountain bike across Asia. In a sense, these things are completely crazy. But if we decide that such ventures are worth doing, we plunge ourselves into a world of physical challenge and in the process, keep some congruence between the body's programming and our contemporary experience.

Physical adventurers are good crazy. By undertaking absurdist outdoor adventures, they keep one foot firmly planted in the Pleistocene, and in the process, keep their wild bodies happy. If we do take on some kind of long-distance, high-intensity challenge, our deep programming suddenly becomes appropriate to conditions. The program "Move when you have to, rest when you can" suddenly becomes functional. To be sure, you'll have fight the elements, but you won't have to fight the deep impulses of your body. There is a kind of peace to this.

If you're willing to plunge yourself into some absurdist, long-distance physical adventure, so much the better. Your body will probably thank you. But of course, not everyone is so inclined, and not everyone has the opportunity to live this kind of lifestyle. Nor is everyone willing to endure the level of risk that comes with these ventures.

If you can't take on an epic fitness challenge, you'll have to rely on your creativity and imagination. Study the ancestral world and look for ways to integrate some primal experience, however brief and fragmentary, into your life. You might not be able to traverse a major wilderness area on foot, but you can probably find a way to traverse local parks, trails and bike paths. Seize these opportunities.

The GoAnimal trail run

This is a highly-adjustable, deeply satisfying physical experience. You'll improve your locomotion skills, pump your cardiovascular system and have a good time doing it. If you're a connoisseur of cardio, you'll love this one.

Start by choosing a hiking trail that includes substantial uphill, several miles at least. There are a lot of good candidates out there to choose from. Throughout the mountainous regions of North American, a great many mountain trails wander up canyons, typically taking 3 to 6 miles to gain a ridge line, pass or viewpoint.

Scout the trail in advance by conventional means. Take a pack with all necessary gear, including maps, water, food and necessary clothing. As you hike, study the basic topography of the trail, especially any stretches of sustained uphill, level, downhill. Also make a mental note of the footing: rocks, mud, creek crossings and so on.

When you return to this trail at a later date, leave the pack and the gear behind. Get an early start and eat a light breakfast. Wear your best trail shoes and a super-light windbreaker or pile jacket. If necessary, wear a small fanny pack. Take a small amount of water if you think it necessary. Don't take a watch; you'll be back long before dark.

When you get to the trail head, start with easy walking for the first few hundred yards or so. This is your warm up. After 10 minutes or so, pick up the pace, then start easy running. If you're really fit, you may be able to run the entire distance, all the way to the pass or overlook. If so, enjoy it.

Most people however, will find several miles of continuous uphill running to be far too ambitious. Nevertheless, you can probably run it in stages. Take it slow at first, concentrating on smooth, easy movement. When running begins to feels too laborious, drop back into a walk. Keep walking until your breathing relaxes, then run again. Alternate your way up the trail with these walk-run cycles. Run a few hundred yards or so, then walk a similar amount. Don't measure the time or distance; simply go by how you feel. Push yourself intelligently, but try to keep your heart rate and breathing rates up.

After a few run-walk cycles, you should be feeling good and ready for a harder push. Now you can run with more intensity. Do longer stretches or pick up the speed. Push until your breath is really heaving, then walk as necessary. If you push too hard, you'll have to stop completely to get your breath, but resume walking as soon as you can. Walk until your breathing and heart rate settle down, but not so far that you cool down completely.

If you're by yourself, you'll be able to customize your pace precisely to what you're capable of. If you're with your friends, you can still make it work. The stronger runners need to be sensitive to the pace of the weaker runners; they may need to walk more than they would otherwise. Nevertheless, they will still enjoy some benefit. If there's a really wide stamina gap in your group, you may need to split up.

In any case, you'll be amazed at how much ground you can cover with this run-walk cycle. Before long, you'll arrive at the pass or the ridge line. When you get there, spend some time taking in the view and enjoying your surroundings. Stay warm, put on your shell and relish the feeling of your thoroughly exercised body. When you're satisfied, head back down.

On the downhill, the challenge is entirely different from what you just experienced. It's not a cardio pump anymore; now it's a skill event. It's important to be conservative. Agility is your primary objective here, regardless of whether you walk or run. If you feel confident, try running stretches of downhill, but don't push your luck. If your footwork gets sloppy or imprecise, slow to a walk. If your knees start to hurt even a little, slow to a walk. Dance your way down the trail with super-precise foot placements.

Remember, this downhill phase is a nervous system challenge. It's easy in the sense that your heart and lungs don't have to work very hard, but it's extremely challenging for the sensory and motor control circuits in your ankles, knees and hips. On the uphill your emphasis was on power and sustainability; on the downhill, your emphasis should be on quality.

No matter whether you're headed uphill or downhill, take a relaxed attitude and pay attention to your surroundings. Allow yourself to be derailed and distracted by beautiful vistas or glimpses of wild animals. By taking on such a substantial physical challenge, you're guaranteed to get a good workout no matter what. If you stop to explore a side canyon or find a beautiful creek, you will loose nothing and perhaps gain a great deal.

Cool down

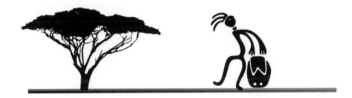

General principles

Let's face it. Integrating exercise into a normal human life is a messy, chaotic and unpredictable business. Sure, we'd like to have a regular schedule, a personal coach and enough free time to do exactly the kind of movement that we really want to do. Unfortunately, few of these things are likely to happen.

Whether you're crafting a training program for prehabilitation, performance or just plain fun, many styles and variations are possible; everyone has a different body, different objectives and different lives. Not only that, unless you are a professional athlete, the reality of daily life tends to upset our most carefully laid training plans. We often have to improvise, throw out the script and work from a set of general concepts. No matter what your style and objectives, these principles will help you get the most out of your effort:

You are responsible for your health and function.

No physician, trainer, or coach can improve your performance, prehabilitate you against injury or rehabilitate you once you're hurt. Professionals can steer you in the right direction and share valuable knowledge, but movement is something that you must do for yourself. There is no free lunch here; the enterprise requires study, attention and effort. If you fail to take responsibility at this level, all the knowledge in the world is worthless.

It's your body.

Each one of us is an genetic individual. We each have unique muscle fiber composition, unique nervous system patterns and unique biochemistry. Our bodies function better in some activities and environments than in others. Science can tell us some things about how the human body works and we can make fairly accurate generalizations about effective training programs. Nevertheless, no one knows your body as well as you do. You know the history of every illness, every injury and every physical success. Listen to the experts and the people that you trust, but in the end, decide what works for you. Be your own animal.

Honor your hominid heritage.

We have more than six million years of hunting and gathering behind us. Imagine the hominid predicament on the open grassland and adjust your movement style accordingly. Take regular trips in the time machine to stimulate your imagination. Do your training outdoors whenever possible and use the power of the natural world to stimulate your senses and movement.

Become a better biped.

A functional gait is crucial to well-being, functional movement and athletic performance. Walk vigorously and often. Study your locomotion and create exercises to improve it. Do lots of hills and train on many different types of terrain. Emphasize diversity, variation, agility and power, not just speed and distance.

Think prehabilitation.

It's far easier to prevent injury than it is to rehabilitate once you're injured. The time to act is now. Think ahead to the probable challenges that your body will face in the future and start designing exercises to strengthen your body to meet them.

Concentrate on fundamental movement skills.

Walk before you run. Run strong before long. Facilitate smooth, controlled movement at the outset. When you master the primary movement, challenge yourself with speed and quickness. Work from the simple to the complex.

Stress integration over isolation.

Teach your body how to operate and move as a single unified structure. You may choose to isolate particular muscles, but do so for a reason. Remember, integration and orchestration are the ultimate goals.

Move often, move vigorously, move gracefully.

Don't get lost in the details of sets, reps, frequency and duration. Just get the movement ball rolling and keep it rolling. Emphasize grace, fluidity and balance. Step lightly and be ready to adjust instantly.

Challenge, but do not punish your body.

Physical stress is therapeutic, but only up to a point; the dose makes the poison. Inflict therapeutic injury upon yourself, but do it in a constructive manner.

Keep a clear sense of oscillation to your efforts.

When you're training easy, train really easy. When you're training hard, train really hard. Be sure to have off days and an off-season. Don't let your efforts plateau at any level. Keep a high level of contrast in your training.

Look for multi-joint, multi-plane movements.

Most functional movements are complex combinations of movement, not isolated to one joint or one plane. In particular, look for spiral, diagonal and figure 8 movement patterns. These movements hold the greatest potential for athletic improvement and fun.

Be an opportunist.

Don't rely on the "official" workout time, place or situation. Fit functional movement and play into the reality of your life. The departure lounge at the airport is your dojo. The rest area along the Interstate highway is your gym. Similarly, be a sloth opportunist. Don't wait for the "official" rest periods in your life–the vacations, the spa, the resort. Fit rest into wherever you can, see how much rest you can get in otherwise unfriendly situations.

Play, dance and bounce whenever possible.

Keep the fun in function. And don't even think about what other people think. Remember, if they won't exercise in public, they're the ones who are dysfunctional, not you.

Set objectives and train to meet them.

Think about what you want out of your body and train precisely for the result that you are trying to achieve. The more specific the detail, the better.

Make every exercise an abdominal exercise.

Challenge your abs to participate in every movement that you do. Whether you're lifting heavy boxes or just picking your socks up off the floor, try to engage all the muscles that surround your torso. After awhile, your body will begin to do this automatically.

Forget what you look like; concentrate on quality movement.

Put your scale in the closet, or better yet, the trash. The quality of your movement is more important than what you look like. If you train for functional fitness, you'll develop a sustainable life of movement. Over the long run, you'll burn more calories and probably lose weight in the process.

Play as if your life depends on it.

In fact, it does. Gravitational, kinetic and resistive stresses are essential to our long-term health and well-being. Without some sort of active, mechanical challenge, the body stops reinforcing the musculoskeletal system and weakness and injury result. Without deep and regular movement, fluids stagnate in the body which leads to all sorts of disorders. Your life literally depends on movement.

Be your own coach.

Be your own best advocate for excellence and well-being. Encourage yourself towards greater performance. Challenge yourself, but never abuse. Strive for excellence, but never forget that the game is only a part of the your total growth and experience. Try as hard as you can, but keep your life well-rounded.

Thanks

Creativity is always tribal. One fellow picks up a stone and flakes off an edge. He uses it to chop down some brush and make a shelter. "Hey, that's a good idea," his friend observes. "But what if we hit the rock at this angle, maybe we could make it just a little sharper. Then we could butcher animals and scrape down the hides for clothing."

And so it goes. After a few generations of refinement, the flakes of stone are razor sharp and with some ingenuity, we figure out how to strap one onto the end of a spear. The tribe enjoys more meat and more warmth in the winter. A few more steps to agriculture, then to industry and so on in a creative explosion. Who shall we give the credit to? The guy who flaked the first stone, his friend who refined the technique or teacher who taught it to his tribe-mates?

Whatever creative success I have had in crafting GoAnimal has been to due in large measure to those who have crafted the stones before me and those who have walked with me along the way. I have flaked off a few chips and made some stones a bit sharper, but I never could have begun without the tribe. I particularly want to thank this fine group of functionalists:

Mom and Dad Forencich, for leading the way and making it all possible. Susan Fahringer and family, for unwavering, extravagant support and inspiration. Sam Forencich and family, for insight, creativity and good cheer. Frank Lindsay, for his active listening and sage counsel. Dr. Dean Edell, for his decades of compassion and intelligence. Tony Yaniro, for his dedication to excellence. Sam George, for his excellent perspective on what it means to be stoked. Gary Gray, for his multi-plane approach to the human body. The departed Carl Sagan, for his relentless honesty and curiosity. Dr. Gerald Eck, for his advice on human origins and the ancestral environment. Vern Gambetta, the coach I wish I'd had. Troy and Anne Corliss, for their artistic encouragement and inspiration. Lysa Rivera, for editing my early work. Fran Tooke, for jumping in with both feet, keeping me on track and heckling me when I needed it. Dennis Schleder, for some truly excellent adventures. The Bainbridge GoAnimal tribe, especially Kyle Elmquist, Ann Summer, Janine Buxton, Teri Shimmin and Carol Wallace. Dustin Gilbert and the good folks at Seattle Vertical World, for hosting GoAnimal classes. Sue Harader and Africa Safari Specialists for arranging my journeys. Johan and Clarenda Visage, for showing me a good time on the Kalahari. Steve Laskevitch and Brian Wood, for their digital mastery and inspired teaching. Colin Fleming for his page layout skills and expertise.

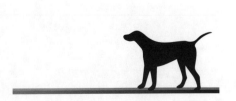